LIVING WELL WITH

Menopause

What Your Doctor

Doesn't Tell You . . .

That You Need to Know

CAROLYN CHAMBERS CLARK, ARNP, EdD, AHN-BC

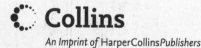

Collins

An Imprint of HarperCollins*Publishers*

FIRST EDITION

ISBN 0-06-075812-0 (pb)

MEDICAL DISCLAIMER

CONTENTS

ACKNOWLEDGMENTS

I want to thank my husband, Anthony Auriemma, who provided unending assistance, freeing me to do my work. Without his love and support, this book would not have been possible.

I want to thank Lisa Shea, founder of BellaOnline, the largest source of information by and for women. She gave me a chance to become an editor at http://Menopause.bellaonline.com. That experience has enriched my life beyond my wildest dreams. It has allowed me to post articles and lead a forum for women going through menopause as well as offer a weekly newsletter updating my subscribers about new menopause information.

This book would not be a reality without my top-notch agent, Bob Diforio, of the D4EO Literary Agency, who is not only a gentleman and a scholar but a caring and efficient man who always responded to my most detailed questions with swift and helpful wisdom. Thanks, Bob.

Thanks to my editor at HarperCollins, Sarah Durand, who not only guided the direction of this book but made working on it a joy. It gives me a tremendous feeling of well-being to know my book has found a home with a publisher that values a wellness and holistic approach.

Thanks to the American Holistic Nursing Association for their encouragement and recognition of my abilities and talents, especially Charlotte Eliopoulus, PhD, RN, past president; Sonja Simpson, RN, MSN, HNC, president; Jean-Ellen Kegler, past executive director; Michael French, communications administrator; members Nancy Oliver, PhD, RN, HNC, and Rory Zahourek, PhD, RN; and Helen Erickson, PhD, RN, AHN-BC, executive director, American Holistic Nurses' Certification Corporation.

A special thanks to all the clients over the years who have asked the important questions and shared what worked for them during the menopause phase of their lives. Their strength, willingness to persevere, and ability to detail their needs and stories have inspired me to produce this book.

Carolyn Chambers Clark

PART I

Menopause and Medical Treatment

1

Introduction

If you're reading this book because you're about to or already have begun menopause, congratulations! You've taken an important step toward understanding the challenges of menopause and acting positively to enter this new phase of life. You've also decided that you want to seize control and take steps to be the happy person you know you can be.

Menopause is one of the most important journeys in your life. It will be thought-provoking, frustrating, confusing, and growth-enhancing. You may start to hate your partner, your kids, your job, your boss, your hair, and even your furniture. This is normal—upsetting but normal.

The idea is to keep in mind that you're not losing control. You're not losing your memory or your mind. Hormonal and other challenging changes are occurring, and as a result, your body, mind, and spirit are reacting. An imbalance has presented you with the opportunity to learn how to weather the effects.

■ My Personal Menopause Journey

I know what you're going through. In my late 30s I started to react with anger and frustration to situations that never used to bother me. In my 40s I began to have trouble sleeping through the night, and I had short periods of panic for no reason at all. My heart would pound as my worries increased. At first I didn't realize that these emotional changes and insomnia were tip-offs that hot flashes, dry skin, thinning hair, and achy joints would soon arrive. As a nurse, I should have known menopause was on its way, but maybe I didn't want to acknowledge it.

As a holistic and wellness practitioner, I didn't even consider taking hormones as my periods waned to a halt. I figured that women had come through menopause for thousands of years before hormone therapy, and they must have discovered ways to manage the changes.

I began to notice I perspired much more and had to wear layers of clothes so that I could peel them off during hot flashes. Having had menstrual cramps, heavy bleeding, bloating, and fatigue for many years, I was secretly happy to turn the page on that phase of my life.

Little did I know that the changes were just beginning. My normal thin and glossy hair grew even thinner and dull. I began to find clumps of it on my bathroom floor. My skin felt dry and itchy despite putting on body lotion. I was gaining weight even though I ate healthy foods. My joints and muscles ached more frequently, and I started to notice short episodes of dizziness. I stopped sleeping through the night, and sometimes it didn't seem as if I slept at all. I would prowl the halls, clicking the TV on and off, hoping to find something to soothe me to sleep. I began to resent the fact that everyone, including my husband, was fast asleep and I wasn't.

I had no idea what to do. The information available at the time was primarily from medical sources and touted taking hormones, which I'd already decided to forego. I knew from my physiology courses what potent substances hormones were, and I didn't want to subject myself to the yet unknown long-term effects.

The prospect of going through this experience alone with no helpful information propelled me into action. I started collecting herb books, holistic books, and anything I could find that even mentioned menopause. It amazed me that no one had collected both the medical and holistic information into one volume. Worse, I could only find a page or two on hot flashes in each source, with only a few suggestions, many of which I'd already discovered or had found didn't work. I constantly shuffled between studies I'd downloaded from the Internet or copied from journals, books, and notes I'd scribbled on pieces of paper.

Added to the mix were my clients, many of whom were entering or were in the throes of menopause and clamoring for information about what to do. They shared their stories with me, and I shared what I was learning from my daily searches for new information.

I had become a vegetarian years earlier, but the beans and rice that had once calmed me now seemed to provoke hot flashes. Ditto the frozen yogurt I'd grown to love. I'd always enjoyed a glass of wine with our Sunday dinner of pasta but found the alcohol now set off horrendous hot flashes.

That's when I knew that even though my lifestyle was healthy, menopause would force me to change the way I lived if I wanted to be more comfortable and more joyful. I changed what I ate, the vitamins, minerals, herbs, and supplements I took, found a new exercise program that worked for me, and began to seek out other holistic practitioners to find what worked for them.

When I talked to my friends and colleagues, I realized I wasn't the only one in the dark. Menopause was not talked about among women the way giving birth and parenting were. It was a dark, secret path that all women eventually took, but one that was not discussed by our mothers, our health care providers, or our friends.

I looked around for ways to connect with more than just the hundreds of women who had come to me for holistic and wellness education. I found bellaonline.com and became the editor for their menopause Web site. As I accumulated articles and brought more and more women to the Web site each month, it sunk in that there are thousands or maybe millions of women out there who could benefit from what I'd learned in my own menopause process and through counseling other women with theirs. That's why I wrote *Living Well with Menopause*. Women deserve to know more about the menopause process and how to cope.

■ Why This Book Is Needed

The U.S. Census Bureau estimates that by the year 2010 more than 20 million women in the United States will be at least 50 years old and menopausal.

Although we all go through a similar process, there are individual variations. Not everyone walks around every night for a year unable to sleep. Not every woman struggles with hair thinning. Not everyone has short periods of dizziness or achy joints and muscles.

There is no way to know which women will suffer from which symptoms. That's why it's important for you to develop your own personal menopause plan.

The medical way is to provide hormones. The root causes of menopause changes are rarely, if ever, explained or addressed. That means millions of women, including you, may ultimately feel alone and unsure about how to proceed.

Now that the World Health Organization has said that hormone replacement therapy is not good for women and research has identified the primarily negative effects of hormones, many doctors are unsure of what to recommend. Some simply shrug as they prescribe an antidepressant. But that isn't the answer now that research has shown that antidepressants may be no better than a placebo (sugar pill) and may increase the risk of suicide.

To top it off, many doctors may not have an answer when you ask, "How can I prevent the conditions that might follow menopause—heart conditions, osteoporosis, and breast cancer?" The unknown can lead to fear. It can make you think you won't be able to recapture your youthful ways, that there is no way to even slow the aging process. You may conclude there are no answers to menopause changes except locking yourself away from life and its joys.

But there are answers. It's just that a typical physician may not have them. Most are too busy to read the holistic and alternative research studies. They're rushing through dozens of patients a day and may barely keep up with their own specialty treatments. They just don't have the time to learn about new approaches except for the new drugs that salespeople bring to their offices.

Even physicians and nurse practitioners who consider themselves experts in women's health rarely venture into the uncharted territory of the menopause process. They can't find the time to really listen to patient complaints and try to find a unique program that each woman deserves.

Studies have shown that women are given inconsistent and incomplete information about menopause. If that isn't bad enough, even female doctors don't have accurate menopause information. One study of 925 female doctors in the Chicago area revealed that only 18% of those surveyed correctly answered seven key questions about menopause. Least knowledgeable were family physicians. The researcher concluded that "physicians may not be an accurate source of information and that there is still a lot of confusion about menopause."

For most women, a holistic and wellness approach is needed. This framework not only deals with symptoms but with the root causes of symptoms. It provides realistic approaches so that you can develop a full-fledged plan that works for you.

When women go to their health care practitioner, the hormone approach might still be pushed, despite the fact that research has shown the possible frightening effects of this route. The media rarely focuses on women's health. You hear information about risk factors related to smoking, being overweight, drinking, and so on, but how often do you hear about the dangers of hormones? You could make the point that menopause is not of interest to that many people. But more than half of the population is facing, has faced, or will one day face menopause.

In a way, the lack of media play is to be expected because menopause isn't a disease like cancer or heart disease. Menopause is a completely normal, natural process, even if the medical community has labeled it a "deficiency of estrogen disease" or "ovary failure disease." Menopause is not a disease, but it does present plenty of challenges.

To make your way through menopause and have a successful life postmenopause, you need an approach that makes you feel good and lets you know that menopause is not the end of life—it's only the beginning. There's no reason to be wrinkled and old, without energy or joy, in pain and depressed. You need to know that menopause is not the dreaded curse of aging. It can be the beginning of your most sexually passionate, creative, and productive phase of life. With the right nutrition, exercise, and attitude, you can look forward to a resurgence of energy and an unexpected opportunity for personal growth.

Trusting your own intuition is really the first step. Don't be like Jill, who couldn't believe she could seize control and develop her own menopause program. She convinced her primary care physician to give her an antidepressant. Although she knew it wasn't working right, she kept taking it, hoping to feel better. When she nearly died from an overdose, she finally realized it was up to her to take a long look at her life and decide on a self-care plan that would work for her. Jill told me:

> *I knew I was going down, down, into a spiral of depression, but I trusted my doctor to save me. Unfortunately, he*

was away the weekend I took too much. Luckily my husband
came home early and found me. Later on I read the research
that antidepressants can lead to suicide. That made me face
the fact that I'd been abused as a child and needed counseling
to get me past that and have a successful menopause.

Finding a practitioner who listens and treats you as an individual
with legitimate ideas and concerns is another important step. I get
hundreds of e-mails a week from women with questions about how
to deal with hot flashes or anxiety or what type of exercise program
will help. They tell me their physicians don't have time to listen to
them and they're not sure why they're taking some of the prescribed
drugs they've been given.

Many of these women have been told they're overreacting when
they complain about gaining weight or having hot flashes. They're
sent home with prescriptions for antidepressants, pain pills, anti-
anxiety medications, and/or estrogen replacement with no discussion of whether these drugs—all of which have secondary effects
that could be harmful—are the best choice, what the underlying
causes of the symptoms might be, and what those causes might
mean.

Candace gained a lot of weight while taking hormone replacement after menopause. She stopped exercising and having sex with
her husband. He eventually left her for another woman. Candace
fell into a deep depression. She told me:

I thought I didn't have anything to live for anymore. Some-
thing stopped me from just hanging it up. Maybe I realized it
was worth staying alive. I started working with a holistic
nurse. She helped me see how my feelings of wanting to be
loved outweighed everything else in my life and how I was
sabotaging myself. Once I realized that, we developed my own
plan for getting me better, and I knew I was on the right track.

Megan had her own set of menopause problems. After the birth of her second child, she was told by her physician that she needed a total hysterectomy, although there was no life-threatening reason for her to have one. As Nancy Lonsdorf, MD, Veronica Butler, MD, and Melanie Brown, PhD, have written in their book, *Women's Best Medicine: Health, Happiness, and Long Life Through Ayur-Veda,* modern medicine is not serving women well.

> *The "art-by-part" system of medicine has led to a number of inappropriate treatments for women ... 27 percent of the hysterectomies were deemed not needed ... several times the rate of hysterectomies performed in European countries. ... Endometriosis, fibroid tumors, prolapsed uterus, even severe menstrual pain are often "solved" by hysterectomy, even though there are safer, less invasive (and less expensive) treatments available.*

Megan hadn't asked for a second opinion about her condition, and she had the surgery. Because of her risk factors for breast cancer, hormone therapy was definitely not an option. Totally unprepared for menopause, Megan went home to take care of her two young children.

> *I had hot flashes and anxiety attacks, and I was up all night, unable to sleep. I was so tired, I didn't see how I was going to cope with the kids. One of them started acting up in school, and the teacher forced us to put him on Ritalin for ADHD [attention deficit hyperactivity disorder]. My husband started working overtime, and I think he was having an affair. I didn't know what to do until I forced myself to take charge of my life.*

■ Why You May Need This Book and What You'll Learn from It

I wrote this book for women like Megan, Candace, and Jill—women who deserve to live well with menopause. I hope this book will help you seize control of your life and find a holistic practitioner with whom you can work, so that you can continue growing and learning.

You need this book if you

- Are going through menopause and feel terrible
- Are going through menopause and haven't even tried to control your symptoms
- Are going through menopause and are trying various methods of symptom control that aren't working
- Have finished with menopause and are losing bone density
- Have finished with menopause and are worried about breast cancer
- Have finished with menopause, have heart disease in your family, and want to take preventive action.
- Know you should quit smoking but haven't been able to
- Are an open-minded health care practitioner who wants to understand and help women going through menopause

Living Well with Menopause will help you go beyond treatments that merely manage symptoms, to discover cutting-edge self-care actions that will not only make you feel better but will help you chart your path for the future and prevent chronic conditions from developing.

■ What You'll Learn from Reading This Book

After reading *Living Well with Menopause* you will:

- Have a tool to assess your menopause symptoms.
- Discover whether hormonal replacement is for you.
- Develop skills to reduce your menopause symptoms.
- Identify underlying causes that could be affecting your menopause symptoms and preventing self-growth.
- Discover resources that can help you.
- Devise a personalized menopause plan that will work for you.

■ About This Book

Living Well with Menopause is different from many other books. This is your book, written by a woman who is not only a holistic practitioner but has been through menopause and understands the confusion and frustrations as well as the joys and potentials.

Living Well with Menopause provides the information about menopause you probably won't find out from your doctor, pharmacy, patient organizations, or in other books on menopause. It provides invaluable insights I've learned from working with clients in my 35 years as a nurse as well as what I've learned from my own menopause. The book includes everything you need to know to live well with menopause—the information, tools, and resources you need to develop a menopause plan and become the best person you can be.

This book gives you what your doctor won't tell you about risk, drugs, and conventional and alternative treatments—what works and what doesn't and the research that explains them. You'll hear the voice of real women who've struggled to pass through menopause and come out whole and happy. Each person in this book wanted to share her own story, ideas, and obstacles with you. I know you will recognize portions of their stories that are familiar, that touch you, that move you to take action yourself. Above all, you'll be convinced you are not alone in your struggle.

■ My Disclaimer

I hope that what you learn from this book will help you decide what menopause plan is best for you and how to find a holistic practitioner to help you implement your plan. Although I've been a nurse since 1964, I am still learning. I seek out information from perimenopausal women and the Internet, speak to health care practitioners, and keep up with the latest research findings. I don't try to go it alone and neither should you. So go find the conventional, alternative, complementary, and holistic practitioners to partner with you in wellness. Don't forget to bring this book along and share it with them.

■ About the Internet

Throughout this book you'll find references to Web sites, articles, and Internet-based resources. If you have access to the Internet, either through your own computer or by visiting your local library and using their free services, visit this book's Web site at http://Menopause.bellaonline.com. The site features a free newsletter, discussion forum, and updated articles based on the latest breaking research. Don't put off your visit to this Web site. It can help you know you're not alone. There are resources and people out there to help you. By choosing to be proactive, you'll feel a surge of personal power and delight. You will be in charge of you.

■ Challenging the Conventional Approach

This book is not meant to stand in opposition to the traditional medical approach. It is the one system that works best in emergencies. Many physicians are caring, able, and healing professionals. They listen to their patients, they seek out new information to better their practices, and they collaborate with holistic practitioners to provide the best possible care. Without medical care, millions of people would die, but the system is not equipped, nor are most of its practitioners, to assist with normal life processes like menopause. For that, you need a holistic, self-care approach fueled by valid information and supported by certified holistic practitioners.

I've worked with many wonderful physicians who keep up-to-date on the latest research and respect the work of complementary and holistic practitioners. I respect them totally. But not all physicians are like them. Some think that only conventional treatments for menopause are effective and that they learned everything they need to know about menopause in medical school. Male physicians may carry stereotypes about women and may not take their complaints seriously. This type of physician scares me and should scare you, too. Remember that health care providers work for you and that you're paying them to carefully listen to your ideas, explain all possible treatments available, and support you in your health care decisions. If they don't listen, explain, and support, you would be well advised to find another medical practitioner who respects you and your opinion.

As you read on, you'll discover that not all medical decisions are based on research. One that wasn't based on good science is hormone replacement therapy, which was once thought to be the perfect answer to menopause. Hormones are now coming under fire as a possible cause of cancer, heart disease, blood clots, gallbladder problems, and liver tumors.

Louise, a 49-year-old CEO of her own construction company,

entered perimenopause and asked me, "Why doesn't my doctor listen to me when I ask questions? I know he's busy, but I have concerns about what's happening to me and I need answers. I answer *my* clients' questions."

I can't speak for her physician or yours, but in this book I try to answer the questions women have raised at my menopause Web site, as clients in my practice, or in the research I've conducted. The opinions of mainstream physicians are well represented in the other books, patient-oriented pamphlets, and Web sites on menopause. Now it's time that the millions of women passing through this natural process called menopause have a chance to be heard and learn how to live well.

2

Menopause: A Natural Process

■ Definitions: Menopause, Premenopause, Perimenopause, Climacteric Postmenopause

Menopause means the end of menses or menstrual periods. The word is derived from the Greek *meno* (month or menses) and *pausis* (pause). Menopause is also known as "the change of life," the end of fertility, and the beginning of freedom.

Whatever you call it, menopause is a unique and personal experience. Menopause is a natural event that happens to every woman at the end of her childbearing years. It is a time of challenges and a time of rebirth when you will have more freedom than ever before to do what you want to do and be who you want to be.

Although some doctors may call a 33-year-old woman in her childbearing years premenopausal, this may not be technically correct. The term *premenopause* refers to the time when you're on the cusp of menopause. Your periods have just started to get irregular.

So far, you haven't experienced any classic menopause changes such as hot flashes or vaginal dryness. You're in your mid to late 40s. If your doctor tells you that you're premenopausal, you might ask how the term is being used.

Perimenopause puts you in the thick of menopausal symptoms. Perimenopause is part of the whole menopause process. Your periods may be erratic, shortened, lengthened, or even vanish. You may have periods that are heavier or lighter or even more painful than usual, which may be puzzling, especially if you were very regular before. You may start experiencing hot flashes and vaginal dryness. If you notice changes in your periods and other body changes, start keeping a diary. This will help you notice any new patterns in your cycle and will be useful information to share with your health care provider as well as to help direct your self-care.

For some doctors, perimenopause represents the period of time that lasts about 4 to 7 years before menopause. It typically occurs around ages 40 to 55 but may occur earlier. Other physicians claim perimenopause begins 2 years prior your last period and ends 2 years after your last menstrual period. These doctors say the average age for the start of perimenopause is 51.

Perimenopause differs from menopause because it occurs earlier than the average age of natural menopause, which is between 51 and 52. Functional eggs are still present in the ovaries. They may be diminishing in number, but they are still available. Your maturing ovaries may not respond as easily as when you were in your 20s. In fact, they may need additional stimulation from the brain and its command centers so that existing eggs may develop, produce estrogen, and undergo ovulation.

While your estrogen level may be low after menopause, during perimenopause the hormone can undergo wild fluctuations. This resulting hormonal roller coaster can result in tremendous hot flashes, sleep disorders, emotional changes, and more.

Although you, your physician, friends, and family may wonder what has gotten into you, what's happening is real. You're not imagining anything. A true physical event has occurred. It's not just that you're stressed, although stress or excitement can worsen the body changes already occurring.

During perimenopause increased levels of estrogen relative to progesterone can produce headaches and irritability. You may think these changes in your menstrual flow signal the beginning of menopause, but the final menstrual period may be at least 5 years away.

At this time, the biochemical pathways for making healthy adjustments in hormonal balance and for producing the steroids secreted and synthesized by the ovaries are still well in place. There are three types of these steroids: estrogens, and androgens, and progesterones.

The *climacteric* lasts from 6 to 13 years and is the stage of your life that encompasses the gradual decline and eventual cessation of ovary function.

The truth is the climacteric is the midstage of life—a time to look back at your life and ponder where you've been, how far you've come, and where you wish to go now that the pressures of childbearing are past. It is a time to grapple with many issues that coincide with but aren't solely related to hormonal function.

Postmenopausal refers to the last third of your life. The range includes women who have been free of menstrual periods for at least one year to women celebrating their 100th (or more) birthday. Once you're postmenopausal, you will be for the rest of your life.

■ Menopause Myths

In some gynecology textbooks menopause is referred to as "reproductive failure" or "ovarian failure." The common teaching was (and in some cases still is) that as we age our ovaries just dry up, shrivel, and become useless. Of course that's not true. Our ovaries don't stop functioning at menopause; they just change gears. We needed high levels of hormones to reproduce, but we don't need them at midlife. Our ovaries still function, but they make less hormones. Menopause is programmed into your life cycle. It's normal and is not a failure on any level.

While the decline is a perfectly normal event, it remains a conventional medical mindset that menopause is a deficiency disease, not a natural process. Endocrinologist and researcher Dr. Jerilynn Prior says:

> *Our culture finds it easy to blame women's reproductive systems for diseases. Linking the menopause change in reproductive capability with aging, making menopause a point in time rather than a process, and labeling it an estrogen deficiency disease are all reflections of nonscientific, prejudicial thinking by the medical profession.*

Calling menopause a disease sets the stage for the pharmaceutical industry to develop drugs to treat it. Stereotypes associated with aging and deep cultural fears are manipulated, and women are led to believe they will lose their attractiveness, dry up, and become brittle once menopause is upon them.

There is no reason for any of these things to occur.

Menopause is not officially classified as a disease, but it's spoken of in the same type of language that's used to describe other medical conditions. We talk about hot flashes, insomnia, and vaginal dryness as menopausual symptoms in the same we say that chest pain and fever are symptoms of pneumonia. Symptoms are anything that bothers you. They don't have to be connected with a disease.

For some reason, we have one kind of thinking about what happens to women and another about what happens to men. If low estrogen is a "disease," then men must really be sick. Another example of this kind of thinking is demonstrated by the fact that men are rarely offered testosterone replacement therapy when their testosterone levels decline.

One of the biggest myths about menopause is that it is a state of deficiency like anemia. Unlike people with anemia who return to health when they get the RDA of iron, postmenopausal women aren't returned to premenopause by taking estrogen.

Why is the term *hormone replacement therapy* even used? It connotes that certain levels of estrogen are "normal" and other levels aren't. Our bodies know when to provide high levels of estrogen and when to provide lower levels.

Another myth is that we're not supposed to live long enough to go through menopause, or if we do, our lives are over. It's true that a few centuries ago women didn't live beyond their 30s, but they were victims of infections and severe illness, or they died in childbirth. If you look at recent history, you'll see there are many vibrant women who have lived through menopause and continue to be productive. If you follow the suggestions in this book, you'll be able have a wonderful life after menopause, too!

■ Hormonal Changes

You're born with about 500,000 egg cells in your ovaries, but only 400 or 500 are mature enough to be released during your menstrual cycle. The other cells gradually degenerate over the years. During your reproductive years, a gland in your brain generates hormones that cause a new egg to be released from its follicle each month. As the follicle develops, it produces *estrogen* and *progesterone*, two sex hormones, which thicken the lining of the uterus. They help prepare the uterus to receive and nourish a fertilized egg should one be available. If fertilization doesn't occur, no fetus develops, and estrogen and progesterone levels drop. The lining of the uterus breaks down and menstruation occurs.

Up until menopause, estrogen helps protect your heart by helping to raise HDL cholesterol (the good kind), which helps remove LDL cholesterol (which is produced in the liver and contributes to the accumulation of fat deposits in your arteries). After menopause, your risk for developing coronary artery disease increases. This is because the veins and arteries that take blood to the heart can become narrowed by plaque.

Estrogen also protects you from bone loss and works with calcium, other minerals, and hormones that help build bone. Your body is constantly building up and laying down bone. Up until about age 30, your body makes more bone than it breaks down. Once estrogen levels start to decline, bone-building does, too. *Osteoporosis* occurs when your bones become too weak and brittle to support normal activities.

An elevated follicle-stimulating hormone (FSH) is the primary marker for the onset of menopause. Your FSH levels will dramatically rise as your ovaries start to slow down. These levels are easily checked through one blood test.

As your ovaries start to shut down, decreased FSH is detected by your hypothalamus, which signals your pituitary gland to secrete FSH and luteinizing hormone (LH). As levels of *estradiol*, the predominant estrogen in your body, fluctuate, your menstrual period length may vary, ovulation may or may not occur, and menstrual bleeding will become irregular. As you near menopause, the effects of the gonadotropins (FSH and LH) result in a complete lack of ovulation and no more periods.

■ How Do You Know You're Going Through Menopause?

When you begin to notice the signs of hot flashes and erratic periods, you'll either suspect the approach of menopause or your health care practitioner will. The FSH test can provide evidence. Your vaginal walls will thin and the cells lining the vagina will not contain as much estrogen. Your health care provider can take a Pap-like smear from your vaginal walls. The results can be analyzed for vaginal changes including the thinning and drying of the vagina. It will help if you keep track of your periods and chart them as they become irregular. Your menstrual pattern will help you and your health care practitioner determine if you are pre- or perimenopausal.

■ Menopause and Pregnancy

Although risk of pregnancy declines each year as you approach menopause, there is always a possibility that you could become pregnant. Your risk of having a child with genetic defects increases in midlife, which is why its important to monitor your periods.

Margie, a 50-year-old administrative assistant, wrote to me about pregnancy. "Can I stop using birth control now that I haven't had a period for four months?"

Many physicians advise that you practice birth control until there's good evidence that you're menopausal, meaning you've had no menstrual periods for a year and are experiencing symptoms such as hot flashes and vaginal dryness. Your physician or nurse practitioner can confirm that you've entered menopause with a blood test.

■ Premature Menopause Through Hysterectomy

Although most women experience "natural" or spontaneous menopause, you can experience menopause due to a medical intervention. Women have asked me, "What happens if I have a hysterectomy?"

I explain there are two types of hysterectomy: partial and complete. In a partial hysterectomy, only the uterus is removed. In a complete hysterectomy, the uterus, fallopian tubes, and ovaries are removed. (The medical term for removal of the ovaries is *oophorectomy*.)

A complete hysterectomy will have a significant impact on hormonal balance because the ovaries are such an important source of hormone production. Even a partial hysterectomy can have a significant effect, first because the uterus plays a role in hormonal balance, and second because in most cases the circulation to the ovaries is impaired enough by the surgery to affect their function.

Surgical removal of both of your ovaries can occur in a procedure known as a *bilateral oophorectomy*. This will trigger menopause at any age. About one in every four American women enters menopause as a result of surgery.

Sheri, one of my clients, asked me about hysterectomy: "I'm having a hysterectomy to remove both my uterus and my ovaries. I'm only 37. Will I go into menopause?"

I told her that hysterectomy with ovarian removal—*bilateral salpingo-oophorectomy*—results in instant menopause. Sheri will no longer have periods, can no longer bear children, and will have many menopausal symptoms right away instead of gradually. This can be quite a shock, so it's best to prepare by talking over strategies with a knowledgeable practitioner. It's also wise to get a second and maybe a third opinion from physicians working in separate practices.

If you have a lot of pelvic pain and you've had several health care practitioners tell you a hysterectomy is necessary, you can still have a good menopause process. If you're worried you'll become more depressed, lose interest in sex, or feel worse after hysterectomy, you may find reassurance in the results of a study conducted by researchers at the Scott and White Clinic in Temple, Texas, which surveyed 178 women (85% were white, and their average age was 40). All had received a hysterectomy for benign, noncancerous conditions such as excessive bleeding, pelvic pain, and fibroids. Participants completed questionnaires on overall and gynecologic health before surgery and 4 and 11 months after, and a depression scale before and 4 months afterward. Most respondents said they felt better physically, emotionally, and psychologically after hysterectomy, regardless of whether they had their ovaries removed or whether they took hormones after surgery. At 4 months, 88% said they felt better. By 11 months, 93% said so. At 11 months, 91% said they were glad they'd had the hysterectomy. At both 4 and 11 months, 85% said they felt less irritable and moody. At 11 months, 66% felt their relationships with others improved. Depression scales remained the same and hormone replacement didn't appear to be a factor. Significantly fewer women reported having pain or discomfort during intercourse. The researchers believed that psychological well-being was influenced by reduced pain and better general health.

If Sheri would have had a hysterectomy but had her ovaries left in place, menopause would not occur because her ovaries would still be able to continue making hormones. Surgical menopause results in a greater decrease in androgen production than does natural menopause and is associated with more pronounced body changes. You'll have hotter hot flashes and more emotional highs and lows. If you're young when you have a hysterectomy, you may still be raising your children. Parenting while experiencing menopause adds additional stress that can affect your energy level and symptoms. All in all, this kind of unnatural menopause can put tremendous strains on you.

■ Other Sources of Premature Menopause

There is some evidence that tubal ligation may bring on menopause or dysfunctional uterine bleeding prematurely. For sure, progesterone levels decrease significantly for at least 6 months following this surgery.

Damage due to radiation to the pelvis, chemotherapy, and certain drugs or medical conditions can also cause menopause to occur earlier than normal. For example, an autoimmune disorder related to poor diet or chronic stress can result in the production of antiovarian antibodies. Chemotherapy, especially with the alkylating agents cyclophosphamide and busulfan, can cause irreversible damage to sex glands. Adding together women who undergo natural premature menopause to those with artificial menopause, approximately 1 in 12 women faces menopause before age 40.

Grieving Premature Menopause

I get e-mails from women all the time who are suffering through premature menopause because they've had hysterectomies. They complain that none of the books they've read have helped them get through the process. Many have young children demanding their attention or husbands who don't understand what they are going through, among other challenges.

Hysterectomy brings on menopause like a tornado descending on an unsuspecting victim and leaves high-powered physical and emotional changes in its wake. Hot flashes can be more intense, vaginal changes greater, emotions more raw. Surgical menopause can be one of the most confusing and difficult times for a woman.

Like other losses in life, surgical removal of your uterus should be grieved. If you don't go through the grieving process, you're liable to retain the emotional and maybe even the physical changes longer.

Resolving your feelings is so very important. If negative feelings about losing your uterus and childbearing ability (and maybe even your ability to have pleasurable sex) aren't resolved, they will continue to affect you. You owe it to yourself, your family, your Maker, and whomever else you touch in life to progress to your highest level of functioning. Find a quiet spot where you won't be disturbed and begin the healing process.

• Invite the sacred. You don't have to be a religious person to invite the sacred. The sacred is anything you revere or respect. Sit comfortably and exhale, emptying yourself of confusion. Breathe in trust. Do this until you feel trust descending. While continuing to breathe, look intently at something intricate and beautiful—a shell, a stone, a flower, a candle flame, or a landscape. Occupy your mind with the word *peace* or *calm*. Feel free to choose your own word. Sense the passage of air through your nose, to your lungs, and out your mouth in peaceful breaths. Invite the sacred to be with you.

• Make a commitment to heal. Rituals are the way we formalize and set aside significant events. Recite or write the following commitment: I _____ (your name) solemnly promise to heal from the sorrow that is with me. I will open myself to messages in my mind, dreams, visions, and fantasies and faithfully record them in a special journal every day. I promise not to judge or censor what I write but to be honest, loving, and accepting of everything I learn. (Be sure to purchase a special journal and write in it daily.)

• Reframe the experience. Put the best possible interpretation, consistent with reality, on the event. What forces drove you toward the decision you made? What would allow you to forgive yourself for your action? What was learned from the event that could be used in your future? Once you have the answers to these questions, you can reframe the hysterectomy as understandable given the factors taking place.

• Release negative feelings. Negative feelings, especially anger and guilt, can confuse and depress you. Use one of the following methods to release negative feelings:

- Picture yourself releasing all your anger and guilt about that event. Find where it's located in your body, turn it into a liquid, and let it run out of your hands and feet and flow far away where it can no longer influence you.
- When you exhale, breathe out resentment, regret, or guilt. When you breathe in, breathe in acceptance.

- Write or speak about your regrets, resentments, or guilt.
- Write or speak about what you appreciate about the event. (Some ideas: Do you appreciate that you did the best you could? Do you appreciate that you came through the experience with the potential for a new life? What else do you appreciate?)
- Write or speak about what you remember or learned by acknowledging what you're grateful for.

- Say good-bye. When you have fully experienced what was and you are open to what will be, you have completed your grieving process. Here are some actions to help you say good-bye:

- Breathe out anguish and breathe in acceptance.
- Find an object you strongly associate with that event or maybe just picture the event in your mind.
- Compose yourself and say whatever you wish you'd said or see yourself doing whatever you wish you'd done.
- Acknowledge how the event has shaped your life and how you plan to dedicate your life to supporting creativity, expression, and intimacy with or in others as a result of your experience.
- Affirm your intention to live in hope for the rest of your life.
- Prepare to release the event by giving whatever blessing you choose, making a pact with the future, and repeatedly saying the word *good-bye*.
- Take note of the vacancy where you once held suffering.
- Sing or play the song "Let It Be."
- Rest. Grieving is exhausting but satisfying work.
- Once you're rested, resolve to consciously choose a life of hope and joy, smiling with pleasure at the small things in life and providing service to others. Peace and pleasure can be yours again. Reach out for it. You deserve it!

■ Perimenopause Changes and Concerns

Perimenopause changes and concerns are not only related to hormonal levels but also to your cultural background, your family history, and your expectations. Smoking can cause an earlier menopause. Emotions and estrogen can also play a role in the stability of your temperature-regulating system and in how your circulatory system functions. Perimenopause changes can range from increased or decreased menstrual bleeding to weight gain.

Breast Cancer and Other Cancers Breast cancer is correlated with too much estrogen, which is often correlated with being overweight. "The more fat you have—fat cells are capable of synthesizing estrogen—the heavier you are, the higher your estrogen levels," says Dr. Paul Tartter, associate professor of surgery at Columbia University. "There's no question that estrogen is the common denominator of most of our risk factors for breast cancer."

Estrogen taken by itself without progestin as part of estrogen replacement can increase your risk of endometrial cancer. Estrogen taken with progestin can increase growth of fibroid tumors in the uterus. Obesity increases estrogen in the blood of postmenopausal women, and high levels of estrogen are a causative factor for breast cancer.

Cold Hands If you have cold hands, your thyroid gland may not be healthy. Hypothyroidism is caused by an underproduction of thyroid hormone. Symptoms include cold hands, constipation, depression, difficulty concentrating, weight gain, muscle cramps, dry and scaly skin, hair loss, and a general feeling of coldness. (Note that many of these symptoms are the same ones women in menopause have.) In fact, about 5 million people in the United States are affected by hypothyroidism, 90 percent of whom are women.

The thyroid gland is your body's internal thermostat. It regulates the temperature of your body by secreting two hormones that control how quickly your body burns calories and uses energy. A cardinal symptom of thyroid dysfunction is cold hands. Reduced circulation due to lack of exercise, reactions to foods, and other factors can also lead to cold hands.

A condition known as *Hashimoto's disease* is believed to be the most common cause of underactive thyroid. In this disorder, the body becomes allergic to thyroid hormone.

Your health care practitioner can measure the thyroid-stimulating hormone (TSH) in your blood to see if your thyroid gland is working correctly. Most endocrinologists believe that TSH levels rise when you're in the earliest stages of thyroid imbalance. An iron absorption test can also be performed. A small amount of radioactive iodine is ingested and an X-ray shows how much of the iodine was absorbed by the thyroid.

A simpler and safer self-test is to take your temperature upon awakening. Place an oral thermometer under your bare arm and sit quietly for 15 minutes. A temperature of 97.6 or lower may indicate an underactive thyroid. Keep a temperature log for 5 days. If your temperature is consistently low, consult your health care practitioner.

Depression, Nervousness, and Irritability   Mood swings and depression may be due in part to alterations in hormones, but they can also stem from causes other than estrogen reduction and other physiological changes taking place at menopause. The results of research on the occurrence of depression as a consequence of menopause are conflicting. It could be that estrogen affects serotonin, and serotonin deficiency is thought to be a cause of depression.

Rebecca was 51 when she came to see me. Here's what she said: "I've finished with menopause, but I still feel so depressed and irritable. Ben tells me I just about bite his head off when he asks a civil question. I feel nervous about things I never used to worry about. When is this going to end?"

Depression and nervousness seem to correlate more directly with aging problems, such as stress in interpersonal relationships and decline in physical health, than with menopause. The only population of menopausal women who show clinically significant depression scores are those who undergo surgical menopause. Dr. Christiane Northrup believes that surges of anger, which are believed to underlie depression, occur because women have sacrificed themselves for their families, but suddenly hormones direct them out of the caregiver role and into an inwardly focused assessment of life and its meaning. Resentments, she claims, not hormones, are what spur women to reexamine the agreements surrounding their relationships with colleagues, friends, and family members.

Taking antidepressants can lead to sex dysfunction according to Dr. Anita Clayton, vice chair of psychiatric medicine at the University of Virginia Health System, Charlottesville. She found dysfunction in at least one phase of the sexual response cycle in more than 95% of women taking antidepressants, with dysfunction least likely to occur in women taking bupropion, although that rate was still very high (70%). With the other antidepressants, dysfunction occurred in the desire phase for 78%–85% of women, in the arousal phase for 82%–87%, and in the orgasm phase for 42%–52%, depending on the medication. Women who experienced dysfunction were most likely to have it in the arousal phase (82%) and in the desire phase (77%). Dysfunction in the orgasm phase was less likely, Dr. Clayton said, with 44% of women experiencing trouble. Dr. Clayton cautioned that percentage may not be accurate because women are "less likely than men to expect to have an orgasm every time they have sex, so if their orgasm rate drops, they might not be as likely to view that as a problem," she said.

Other factors may come into play for women like Rebecca who have a natural menopause process. Facing the empty nest as children leave or the revolving door as they return, caring for an elderly relative, or a sense of unfinished business in their lives can overtake women at menopause and contribute to mood swings and depression.

Rebecca's son, Charles, had just graduated from college and couldn't get a job. When he moved back in and got into arguments with her husband. Rebecca's stress increased. I told her the stress she was feeling was real and anyone would feel depressed in her situation. After three family therapy sessions. Charles and his father started to work things out between them, Rebecca's stress decreased, and so did Rebecca's irritability and depression.

Other situations that could lead to depression and/or anxiety at this time include:

- Having been depressed during your lifetime about other situations and not having learned how to grieve and deal with anger
- Feeling negative about menopause and getting older
- Severe menopause symptoms
- Smoking
- Physical inactivity
- Not being happy in a relationship or not being in a relationship
- Being unemployed
- Lack of money
- Low self-esteem
- Not having the family or friend support you need
- Regrets that you can't have children anymore

This book of self-care and wellness procedures may be especially helpful because many of the medications used to manage depression have undesirable side effects including:

- Weight gain
- Vaginal dryness
- Orgasm disruption

- Loss of sexual desire
- Fatigue
- Lethargy
- Depression that leads to suicide in rare cases

Dizziness A primary cause of dizziness during perimenopause and postmenopause is iron deficiency. Obtaining sufficient dietary iron is one solution. Read more about this in chapter 4.

Fatigue If you're losing sleep due to night sweats and hot flashes and you're gaining weight and on an emotional roller coaster, no wonder you feel fatigued. Top that off with an imbalanced thyroid and you'll be very low on energy.

Hair Loss/Thinning Hormonal changes, inadequate diet, insufficient exercise, how you treat your hair, and aging factors (such as the medications you take and genetics) can lead to hair loss and thinning.

Headaches The problem with taking conventional drugs for headache is the rebound effect. This insidious increase of headache frequency is associated with the use of headache medication. The overuse of headache drugs can lead to more headaches and even more when you attempt to discontinue the drug.

If you suffered from menstrual migraines, you may get a reprieve, or you may get even more headaches. Potential triggers for headaches include food, alcohol, lack of fluids, stress level, taking hormones, and amount of sleep.

Exercise and sexual activity may diminish your headaches. By keeping a record of what you eat, stressful situations you encounter, and medications you take, you may be able to identify what's setting off your headaches. If you are taking hormones, speak to your health care practitioner about trying a different kind or brand.

Heart Disease   Heart and blood vessel disease is correlated with decreased estrogen. As estrogen's protective effect recedes, increased "bad" cholesterol and an unfavorable lipid profile may result. High plasma total cholesterol is believed to be a risk factor for coronary artery heart disease. A favorable lipid profile includes an increased high-density lipoprotein (HDL) cholesterol and a decreased low-density lipoprotein (LDL) cholesterol.

Your cholesterol level is not only determined by what you eat. Your body produces its own cholesterol. LDLs are produced in the liver and carried to the peripheral tissues, where they provide energy for heart muscle. Estrogens protect against heart disease by lowering levels of LDL cholesterol and raising the concentration of HDL cholesterol. The net effect is to prohibit fat from accumulating and to improve blood flow to the arteries to the heart.

In the United States, 27% of all women aged 20 to 74 have total cholesterol levels higher than 240 mg/dL. As you age, you have a reduced ability to remove the LDL "bad" cholesterol from your body. Within 6 months after menopause, your total cholesterol levels could increase by 6%. By 2 years postmenopause, LDL cholesterol levels could increase by 10% and HDL cholesterol could decrease by the same amount. A 1% increase in plasma total cholesterol or LDL is believed to increase your risk of coronary artery disease by 2%. A 1% decrease in HDL is believed by some experts to increase your risk of coronary artery disease by 2% to 4%.

But it's not only high LDL cholesterol that puts you at risk of heart disease. If you're overweight and don't exercise, your risk for coronary artery disease rises. Seventy percent of heart disease in obese women and 40% of heart disease in all women is attributed to being overweight, which is preventable.

Smoking is the single highest preventable risk factor for heart and blood vessel disease in women. Cigarette smoking is directly responsible for 21% of deaths from heart and blood vessel disease and for 50% of all heart attacks before age 55. It is the nicotinic release of catecholamines that stimulates the nervous system and increases plasma levels of LDL cholesterol. Smokers are known to have an unfavorable plasma lipid profile, including increased levels of total cholesterol and triglycerides and decreased levels of HDL cholesterol. Cigarette smoking can eliminate the protective effect of estrogen on your heart and blood vessels and is associated with a risk of early menopause. (See chapter 6 for information on how to stop smoking.)

Hot Flashes Vasomotor flushes or hot flashes are characterized by sweating and an intense feeling of heat around the head and neck. Hot flashes can be problematic for several months, several years, or even 10 years or more. When they create sleep deprivation, depression can result.

In Nancy Pickard's novel *Twilight,* the character Jenny Crain has a conversation with a friend about hot flashes. She says, "Jenny, I want you to know that hot flashes can be wonderful." Jenny can't believe her ears and she gulps. Her friend continues. "Really. This is the only time in my life I've ever been warm. I get up to go to the bathroom in the middle of the night, and my feet aren't freezing. Sometimes I lie in bed and think, oh, this is so nice."

Hot flashes or hot flushes are not magical changes. They can result when estrogen is low and an imbalance occurs. They are a way your body cools you off. The disruption in temperature control in your hypothalamus is associated with a sharp rise in blood levels of epinephrine, a potent stimulator of heart function. Some experts believe hot flashes and profuse perspiration are a result of an alteration in blood vessel control in the periphery of the body. This theory explains why women commonly report that their heart pounds. In fact, clinical measures show that heart rate does increase during a hot flash. Because the heart is beating faster, blood pressure can rise, and headache and dizziness can occur. While core temperature doesn't increase, you could feel intense warmth throughout your upper body, with flushing of the neck, face, and chest, and in some cases, profuse perspiration followed by chills. The chills are your body's way of trying to conserve body heat.

You could be part of the majority of perimenopausal women who suffer from hot flashes. Only about 15% to 25% of these hot flashes are severe or frequent (more than 10 a day). The duration of a hot flash varies from a few seconds to minutes. The average number of hot flashes is 10 a day, with the majority occurring at night, but frequency also varies from person to person and even in the same woman.

When pressed, the American Medical Association admitted that only 5% of women suffer any major menopausal problem, but because of increasing advertising and medical research paid for by drug companies, many women are being brainwashed into thinking that temporary discomforts are serious. Other experts believe that expecting problems at menopause can lead to actual difficulties. For sure, getting uptight about hot flashes can increase them because one of the common triggers for hot flashes is stress.

The medical community has not conducted any controlled prospective trials on the menopause experience of healthy women who exercise regularly, eat a proper diet, don't smoke, and lead a healthy lifestyle. This is probably because the cultural focus in the United States is on menopause as a problem and even as a disease.

Some cultures where menopause is not a problem have been studied. Anthropologist Ann Wright found that traditional Navajos exhibited few symptoms, and unlike our society, postmenopausal women gained increased decision-making power and respect as they grew older. Her study suggested that menopause symptoms are related to psychological stress, not physical stress. Kung women in Africa have increased status after menopause. There isn't even a word for hot flash in their language. Either Kung women don't experience hot flashes or maybe they accept them as normal and don't view them in a negative light. In contrast, 65% to 90% of American women can experience hot flashes, and a large number complain of vaginal dryness and loss of interest in sex.

Insomnia/Sleep Problems   Melatonin, a hormone secreted by the pineal gland, helps set your biological clock, which dictates the smooth running of your body on a daily basis. When this mechanism falls out of sync, insomnia is one result. Melatonin tends to decline with age. Recent evidence suggests that melatonin levels are lower if you're overweight and postmenopausal.

Night sweats can interfere with efficient sleep patterns, and so can tight muscles, hot flashes, and other menopause changes. All can lead to daytime fatigue, irritability, memory loss, nervousness, and anxiety. Lack of vitamins and minerals can also interfere with sleep, as can emotional reactions.

Itchiness   Itchiness can be due to dry skin, nutritional deficiencies, or lack of estrogen.

Joint and Muscle Pain   Joint and muscle pain can be due to deficiencies in vitamins, minerals, or fluids. If you're not eating foods that contain the vitamins and minerals you need or taking a good multivitamin and a good multimineral, and if you're sweating a lot due to hot flashes or night sweats, you may need additional nutrients and water (see chapter 4).

Memory Loss and Foggy Thinking   Memory loss and foggy thinking may be related to estrogen reduction, but they may not. Estrogen may stimulate the growth of nerve cells and increase the levels of acetylcholine, an important transmitter of nerve messages in the brain. One study showed that women who suffered surgical menopause and who were given estrogen after surgery had better scores on tests of memory and abstract reasoning compared to other women who were given a placebo (sugar pill).

Other experts maintain that memory loss and fuzzy thinking are part of normal development and are usually self-limiting. Studies have provided evidence that thinking and memory loss occur no more frequently at menopause than at other times in a woman's life.

Some researchers have reported that both chemotherapy and tamoxifen (an antiestrogen drug with many adverse reactions) can cause fuzzy thinking. Researchers at Rush University Medical Center in Chicago found that forgetfulness is not caused by menopause. In fact, the hormone supplement industry was built partly on the premise that estrogen pills could keep women's minds sharp. That idea has been challenged by this research. The participants were not taking hormone supplements, which were recently linked to an increased risk of dementia in older women. Instead, the women were given two standard memory tests every year and were followed for an average of a little more than 2 years. Scores declined only slightly for postmenopausal women but no more than would be expected with normal aging, according to Peter M. Meyer, the lead researcher and a biostatistician. The researchers claimed that if women are sometimes forgetful, it is probably not because of any harmful hormonal changes in their brains but because they are busy, distracted, and stressed out dealing with the ordinary pressures of midlife.

Fuzzy thinking can also be due to a sluggish thyroid, which in turn can be caused by deficiencies of zinc, selenium, and copper. As you age, your digestive enzymes and hydrochloric acid are reduced. Both are critical for the proper breakdown of food and the nutrition your mind and body need. All these situations can affect your ability to think clearly.

Menstrual Bleeding Bleeding during perimenopause can be erratic and scary. You think you're approaching menopause, then suddenly you have a heavy-flow period.

Hormonal fluctuations lead to fluid retention, which affects circulation, reducing the amount of oxygen reaching your uterus, ovaries, and brain. Heavy marijuana use decrease the amount of hormones released, which can cause irregular bleeding. Eating red meat and dairy products may cause or contribute to hormonal imbalance. Unstable blood sugar levels are an important factor, too.

Food allergies, vitamin and/or mineral deficiencies, and depressed mood can also lead to hormonal fluctuations.

Think of your body as a unit. When one part gets out of sync, the whole process can get sidetracked. The more balance you can bring to your body, mind, and spirit, the easier your menopause will be.

Osteoporosis   Osteoporosis is one of the most common and disabling conditions affecting women after menopause. The amount of bone in your skeleton is a function of your genetic inheritance, how much calcium you take in, your vitamin D consumption, your peak amount of bone mass, your rate of bone mass loss, and what drugs and medications you take.

A 2003 study in the *Archives of Internal Medicine* examined the risk of bone fractures in more than 8,000 women over age 65. All of the women were taking some type of medication that affected the nervous system, such as the most commonly prescribed antidepressants. Over a period of 5 years, researchers found that the women had a significantly greater chance of sustaining fractures compared to women who didn't take these types of drugs. When the data were broken down more specifically, women who took antidepressants were found to be 70% more likely to suffer disabling hip fractures. Researchers suspect that reduced alertness prompted by the drug use was to blame for the higher incidence of fractures.

Some experts believe the principal determinant of skeletal status is your ovary function. The precise way that estrogen influences bone remodeling is not known, but specific receptors for estrogens have been identified in cells of bone tissue.

Estrogen reduction may have a negative influence on your ability to use calcium. Calcium absorption through the intestine decreases and calcium loss from the kidney increases, resulting in an increased use of skeletal calcium to maintain calcium in the blood. Other factors that increase your risk for osteoporosis include:

- Taking glucocorticoids (cortisone, Decadron, Dexameth, Dexon, Cortef, Medrol, Delta-Cortef, Prelone, Deltasone, Orasone, Panasol, Meticorten, Aristocort, Atolone, Kenacort)
- High consumption of caffeine, animal proteins, and sodas
- Alcohol consumption
- Cigarette smoking
- Prolonged bed rest or lack of weight-bearing exercise
- Taking thyroid and/or parathyroid hormones
- Family history of osteoporosis

During the climacteric, women show a 2% to 5% loss in bone mass a year, but reduced estrogen is not the only factor involved because women lose up to 50% of their total bone mass before menopause. From the ages of 25 to 34, between 6% and 18% of women exhibit low bone density. Hip fracture rates are also high before menopause even occurs. Other factors that can lead to osteoporosis include smoking, excessive alcohol intake, a mother who suffered severe osteoporosis, lack of exercise, a high-fat, high-carbohydrate diet, never having given birth, feeling depressed, a history of ovulatory disturbances, low body fat, and deficiencies in calcium, magnesium, and other minerals.

Sex Drive Reduction and Intercourse Discomfort It's on the TV screen and in the movies. Sex is everywhere except in the bedroom. Sociologists at the University of Chicago asked 3,159 women and men chosen to represent the larger U.S. population about their sex lives. They found that 43% of the women and 31% of the men reported some persistent sexual dysfunction such as inability to become aroused or to achieve orgasm.

If you were interested in sex and enjoyed intercourse when you were younger, you'll probably feel the same way after menopause. If you were never able to achieve orgasm, you may be able to now that you can relax and not worry about becoming pregnant. You may never have explored your body sufficiently or participated in enough foreplay to become aroused.

Tammy, a 48-year-old engineering student, confessed that although she was having hot flashes and other signs of menopause, she had never had an orgasm and wondered what to do about it. We started with basic anatomy and sexual information.

The opening to your vagina is shielded by the mons veneris (the fatty tissue at the base of your abdomen that becomes covered with hair at puberty), the labia (folds of tissue that extend downward on either side of the vagina), and the clitoris (located at the top of your vulva where the labia meet; it becomes erect when you're sexually aroused). The external organs of generation in the female are the mons, veneris, the labia majora and minora, the clitoris, the meatus urinaries or opening to the bladder, and the opening to the vagina. The term vulva or pudendum includes all these parts. Between the clitoris and vagina is your urethra, a 1½-inch passageway that leads to your bladder, where urine is stored.

The process that takes place in your body during sexual intercourse remains the same no matter what your age. It consists of four stages:

1. *Excitement.* In response to touch, visual images, or fantasy, cells in your vagina and nearby glands begin to secrete lubrication fluid, and your heart rate and blood pressure may rise. The clitoris fills with blood and enlarges, your nipples become erect, and your breasts may increase in size. Your vagina lengthens and expands while the fleshy lips that surround your vaginal entrance swell. You may develop a rosy flush that begins over the upper abdomen and spreads over the breasts.

2. *Plateau.* Tissues in your vagina continue to swell. Your clitoris retracts under the folds of tissue that surround it.

3. *Orgasm.* If orgasm occurs (and it doesn't happen each time you have intercourse) a series of intense and pleasurable contrac-

tions takes place in the muscles of your vagina, uterus, and sometimes your rectum. The number of orgasmic contractions ranges from 3 to 5 per minute to 8 to 12 per minute.

4. *Resolution.* In the next 30 minutes, muscle tension decreases and the swelling of tissues subsides. Your heart rate and blood pressure return to normal.

While age doesn't alter these steps, reduced interest in sex and intercourse discomfort after menopause can be related to vaginal dryness, irritation, and thinning, which can be due to decreased estrogen levels. Depression and anxiety can also interfere with sexual interest. During the climacteric, thinning of the walls of the vagina can lead to dryness, infections, burning, itching, pain with intercourse, discharge, and occasional bleeding unless you take steps to counter these changes.

> *Alice, a 49-year-old woman, was nearing menopause. She called me when she started having heavy bleeding, wondering if she should be concerned. Here's what I told her. "Changes in bleeding are normal as you near menopause. The decline in your body's estrogen levels can cause tissues lining your vagina to become thin, dry, and less elastic. This lining can become broken or easily inflamed and bleed. It can also become injured during sex or even during a pelvic exam."*

Once you've reached menopause, you should report any bleeding that you have to your health care practitioner. Uterine bleeding after menopause could be a sign of fibroids, a hormonal imbalance, or noncancerous growths in the lining of the uterus, among other health problems.

As estrogen decreases, vaginal secretions are altered in quantity and composition. The possibility of vaginal infection increases because your normal protective lactobacilli that assist with digestion decrease, permitting overgrowth of organisms from the vagina and surrounding area. Burning and irritation can be caused by a chronic discharge because of the change in the composition of secretions. Itching can occur because of the thinning and inflammation of the vagina.

The cells of the vagina and urethra contain high concentrations of estrogen receptors. Within 5 years of estrogen decrease, changes occur in the vagina, urethra, and bladder. Since estrogen increases blood flow in arteries, when estrogen decreases, there is a decrease in blood flow to the vagina and vulva, resulting in atrophy of the vaginal walls, flattening of lubrication glands, and loss of water-retaining ability. These changes can reduce lubrication and shorten and narrow the vaginal wall, which can lead to pain during intercourse.

Between 30% and 50% of women complain of a problem in one or more aspects of sexual functioning, probably due to reduced vaginal lubrication, atrophy of the vagina, and frequent infections. In a study of 887 menopausal women, pain during intercourse was the most common sexual problem, followed by decreased sexual desire, partner problems or dysfunctions, vaginal spasms, and lack of orgasms. The researchers found that the lower the level of estradiol, the greater the discomfort during intercourse.

Low estradiol levels correlate with decreased blood flow to the vagina. This makes vaginal engorgement, which is necessary for comfortable sexual intercourse, impossible. A catch-22 syndrome can develop: discomfort with intercourse, apprehension about intercourse, decreased frequency of intercourse due to fear of pain. Women who stop having intercourse, whether it's due to loss of sexual desire, discomfort during intercourse, or another reason, develop even more vaginal thinning than women who continue to be sexually active.

Some experts claim that loss of interest in sex is not related to estrogen levels and shouldn't necessarily occur at menopause. They present statistics to show that more than 40% of menopausal women report no decline in sexual interest. Less than 20% report any significant decline, but women who've had oophorectomies, hysterectomies, chemotherapy, or radiation usually have a loss of interest in sex.

Skin Problems Wrinkles are largely due to cross-linking of proteins. You can reduce them by retarding oxidative damage and free-radical destruction. Dehydration is another cause of dry skin. If you don't drink enough water, your skin can look dry and saggy. Skin thickness declines just as bone density does after menopause. To have beautiful skin, you must eat healthy foods and drink enough water to feed your skin, and use products that protect it.

Urinary Symptoms Urinary symptoms can include difficulty urinating, frequent and urgent urination, frequent nighttime urination, dribbling of urine, and frequent urinary tract infections. Some experts claim these symptoms will worsen over time.

Other experts claim vaginal and urinary complaints are highly individual and subjective. A physician's diagnosis of atrophic vaginitis may not always be accompanied by symptoms and vice versa. Urinary frequency and bladder infections sometimes are associated with vaginal thinning and thinning of the urinary apparatus but not always.

Weight Gain If you don't exercise daily and don't watch what you eat, it is easy to gain weight after menopause because you are losing muscle—another reaction to hormonal changes. Don't talk yourself into thinking weight gain is okay. Being overweight puts you at risk for even more chronic conditions. Obesity contributes to high blood pressure, which is a significant and independent risk factor for heart disease.

Being overweight is also a significant factor in diabetes, which accelerates the laying down of fat in your blood vessels and decreases blood flow through the heart. High blood pressure, obesity, and diabetes often occur together and can contribute to an overall high-risk profile postmenopause. (See chapters 4 through 9 for more information on how to lose weight and/or prevent weight gain.)

3

Medical Treatment

Medical treatment for menopause includes hormones and surgery. Being able to communicate with your medical provider and receive adequate answers to your questions are also part of treatment.

■ What Women Say About Menopause

I surveyed 50 menopausal women in 1999–2000, asking them about their menopausal symptoms, what they did to relieve them, their self-image, how their current self-image compared to pre-menopause, what information they needed to have a more comfortable menopause, and anything else they wanted to tell me.

Some of my study participants questioned the use of hormones even before the studies started pouring in about possible harmful effects. One 50-year-old woman was in perimenopause. She complained of hot flashes, weight gain, muscle pain, muscle spasm, dribbling urine, pain with intercourse, and night sweats. When surveyed about what information she needed to be more comfortable about menopause, she replied, "Risks versus benefits of hormone replacement treatment. Right now I'm using the 'Mother Nature' method. My doctor prescribed hormones but didn't tell me anything about what to expect. When my breasts started to hurt, I bloated up, and got depressed. I threw the bottle out."

■ Hormone Treatment

Hormone treatment or therapy (HT) is also called hormone replacement therapy (HRT). HT or HRT refers to the use of prescription drugs to "replace" ovary-produced hormones. There are several kinds of hormones, but estrogen and progesterone are the two main ones.

Estrogen

The medical theory behind female hormones is that women should be producing estrogen and not to do so is a disease. For many years, physicians, nurse practitioners, and physician assistants have prescribed estrogen replacement therapy (ERT) to relieve menopausal symptoms. Because taking a drug that includes only estrogen raises the risk of endometrial cancer (cancer of the lining of the uterus), only women who do not have a uterus can take estrogen (ERT) alone safely. ERT is usually taken by mouth, absorbed from a skin patch, or applied as a vaginal cream.

In the 1940s, estrogen was first offered to menopausal women. Harvested from the urine of pregnant mares and made into a pill called Premarin, it was designed to be given to women between ages 45 and 55 in the throes of menopause. Although Premarin is a natural estrogen produced in a laboratory, it is potent and may cause metabolic changes in the liver. Estrogen from horses should probably not be used by women who are obese, who smoke, or who suffer from high blood pressure, high cholesterol, or varicose veins.

In the 1960s, hormones as a panacea for a variety of ailments began to gain hold. While early studies suggested hormones prevented heart disease and improved quality of life, much of the research used questionable methods, did not indicate the strength of the pills, and did not address whether they contained just estrogen or a combination of estrogen and progestin, another hormone (a synthetic form of progesterone). Most of these studies were observational in nature and did not contain the gold standard of research: a relevant control group similar to the study group but composed of women not taking the hormone under study.

According to Dr. Susan Love, at SusanLoveMD.org, it was Dr. Robert Wilson, a New York gynecologist, who ignited the fervor for hormones in 1966 in his book, *Feminine Forever,* when he branded menopause as a "horror of living decay" that demanded aggressive medical treatment. Other physicians took up the cry. His son, Ronald Wilson, said that drug makers gave Dr. Wilson his platform and that he was underwritten by the Wyeth drug company.

There are three types of estrogen: estrone (E1), estradiol (E2), and estriol (E3). Estradiol and estrone are the two most commonly used in hormone therapy. They are available in a wide variety of preparations, from transdermal patches to oral forms. Ideally, the preparation should match your body's hormones. It should include a combination of estrone and estradiol from a formulary pharmacy— for example, Estrace and the Estraderm or Climera patch—all estradiol, or a type of estrone such as Orthoest.

Estrogens used in conventional estrogen replacement therapy are estradiol and estrone, but both have been implicated in breast cancer. Being overweight and taking estrogen can be a double whammy. The scenario works this way: weight gain creates fatty tissue, which makes estrogen, and estrogen can help breast cancer grow. Dr. Paul Tartter, associate professor of surgery at Columbia University, says,

"There's no question that estrogen is the common denominator of most of our risk factors for breast cancer."

A February 2004 study by the American Cancer Society found that postmenopausal women who gained 20 to 30 pounds after high school graduation were 40% more likely to get breast cancer than women who kept the weight off. The risk doubled if a woman gained more than 70 pounds, according to Heather Spencer Feigelson, senior epidemiologist with the Cancer Society. Lean, postmenopausal women not taking hormones had the lowest cancer risk.

If you have had breast cancer or an estrogen-associated cancer, are overweight, or have concerns about breast cancer, you aren't a suitable candidate for conventional ERT. An alternative is estriol, a somewhat weaker estrogen. Estriol does not cause changes in the lining of the uterus. Taking progestin in addition to estrogen doesn't reduce breast cancer risks.

According to Dr. Donnica L. Moore, president of Sapphire Women's Health Group in Neshanic Station, New Jersey, the controversy over the link between breast cancer and estrogen replacement will lead to the development of drugs such as selective estrogen receptor modulators (SERMs) because of their ability to act like estrogen in some tissues but not in others. The Food and Drug Administration has granted market clearance to raloxifene (Evista) to provide a "useful alternative" to estrogen, but it is not a substitute. Although raloxifene may reduce the risk of breast cancer by more than 50%, it can produce hot flashes and leg cramps. A rare but serious side effect are blood clots in the veins, which occur at a rate similar to that seen with estrogen. It is not to be used by women who are or may become pregnant.

■ Physician Misuse of HRT

A drug marketed as Prempro had sales soaring to $888 million globally by 2001. Prempro and other hormone replacement medicines were widely prescribed as a way of preventing heart disease and restoring quality of life, even though the Food and Drug Administration only approved their use for hot flashes and the prevention of osteoporosis. This happened because physicians are allowed to stray outside the drug's approved purpose in a practice called off-label use. As a result, physicians began prescribing the pills to erase wrinkles and boost mental functioning in women.

By the 1990s, 6 million American women were taking combination hormone replacement therapy. Many took it only for a few months to ease menopause changes, whereas others took it for years thinking it would slow the advance of aging.

"Instead of examining the data," Dr. Judith K. Ockene, chief of preventive and behavioral medicine at the University of Massachusetts Medical School in Worcester and a principal investigator of the Women's Health Initiative, said, "if they [physicians] see that other physicians are doing something, then it adds to their decision-making as to whether to do it."

■ HRT and Uterine Cancer

Hormone therapy suffered its first round of scientific setbacks in 1975 when researchers reported that women using estrogen alone ran a significantly higher risk of developing uterine cancer. A search for an alternative was sought, and the result was a pill that combined estrogen with progestin, which negated the cancer threat.

After 50 years of trial and error, it is well known that estrogen stimulates growth of the inner lining of the uterus (endometrium), which sheds during menstruation. This growth may continue uncontrollably, resulting in cancer.

There are unpleasant side effects of progestin that often discourage women from continuing HRT, including breast tenderness, bloating, abdominal cramping, anxiety, irritability, and depression. Even with newer types of HRT, such as taking progestin for only the first 12 days of the month, in many cases, monthly bleeding is replaced with irregular bleeding. It may take 6 months or longer until bleeding finally stops.

■ HRT Linked to Breast Cancer, Blood Clots, and Heart Disease

In 2003, the Women's Health Initiative found that a women's risk of heart attack rose by 81% in the first year of hormone therapy. The study of more than 16,000 women was halted three years early. Conclusions were so damning from the Women's Health Initiative, that the National Institutes of Health put an early halt to the review once researchers found that combined hormones increased a woman's risk of breast cancer, blood clots, and heart disease. Further results found that not only did the combination hormone pill not improve the quality of life, it doubled the risk of dementia in women 65 and older.

Since then, other researchers have provided similar bad news for hormones. A study released by the National Cancer Institute found that the increase in breast cancer risk is especially high for overweight women and is "largely the result of the increase in taking estrogens, particularly bioavailable estradiol." A 2003 study in the *International Journal of Cancer* stated that using the combined estrogen-progestin hormone replacement therapy is associated with an increased risk of lobular breast cancer and invasive ductal cancer. The researchers concluded that being overweight/obese is associated with ductal cancer, while hormones and oral contraceptives are related to an increased risk of invasive lobular breast cancer. Drinking one or more alcoholic drinks daily and taking postmenopausal hormones doubles your risk of breast cancer.

In 2000, a Norwegian study found that women who had a previous leg clot had an increased risk for additional clots if they took HRT. A study paid for by the British government of one million British women found a higher death rate from breast cancer among those who took combination hormone therapy than those who did not use it or took estrogen alone. The risk of developing breast cancer was double for those taking estrogen-progestin compared to those not taking hormones. For those taking only estrogen, the increased risk was 30%. This is the largest study to show the effects of hormones on breast cancer. Findings also strengthened recent recommendations against using long-term combination hormone therapy to prevent chronic conditions like bone fractures from osteoporosis.

One comforting finding was that the risk for breast cancer declined gradually after women stopped hormone therapy. Five years after quitting, women faced no greater risk than those who had never taken HRT. Dr. Marcia L. Steanick of Stanford University commented, "It looks like the longer you use hormones, the worse off you are."

Dr. Ford of the National Cancer Institute said the British study supported findings reported in June 2003 suggesting that combination hormone therapy led to more aggressive cancers that were detected at a more advanced stage than among women not taking such therapy. Combined therapy also increased the percentage of women with abnormal mammograms, according to a study published in the *Journal of the American Medical Association.*

■ HRT Withdrawal Increases Bone Loss

A study published in *Bone* in 2003 found that the rate of bone loss after withdrawal of HRT was significantly greater than in postmenopausal women who never took HRT. The researchers concluded, "In postmenopausal women who have been on HRT for 6 years, cessation of treatment results in a rapid increase of bone turnover loss similar to early postmenopausal women during the subsequent 4 years and greater than untreated women of the same age."

■ HRT Increases Gallstone Formation and Arthritis

Other studies also identified problems with the use of estrogen. A 2003 study in *Menopause* found that ERT increased the chances of gallstone formation. Another study in the same journal found that taking HRT for 5 years or less did not preserve bone or significantly reduce fracture risk in later years. A study published in *Maturitas* in 2003 concluded that while breast-feeding may protect against hand osteoarthritis, current or past use of hormone replacement therapy was significantly associated with increased prevalence and severity of hand osteoarthritis.

A 52-year-old participant in my menopause study sought medical help in her 30s for mood swings and irregular periods. She told me:

> *I was dismissed by the female physician who told me "Read some books." I went to another physician who placed me on heightened levels of progesterone (shots), which somehow masked my hot flashes, insomnia, and depression. Years later, another physician was alarmed at my high level of progesterone. Over the next three years, he gave me a regime of natural estrogen, progesterone, and testosterone. A specialist working with my gynecologist continued to elevate my estrogen in the attempt to create a normal period. As a result, a few years ago I developed a precancerous state resulting in the need for a complete hysterectomy. Now I have arthritis in my*

*hands and my doctor says I may need to have my gallbladder
out. Needless to say, I'm livid. I've endured so much bleeding
and feel depleted. My only regret is that I had to endure the
pain and frustration of feeling helpless for quite some time.
Hopefully women are more educated as to the options available.*

■ HRT Linked to Asthma, Diabetes, and Parkinson's Disease

Studies have shown that HRT is associated with an increased rate of
newly diagnosed asthma. Women with diabetes are at an increased
risk for death from all causes, including heart disease, when they
take HRT. Drinking caffeinated drinks also increases the risk of
Parkinson's disease among hormone users.

■ Other HRT Cautions

A 2004 editorial in *The Lancet* warned long-term users of combination hormones to stop them as soon as possible, but physicians
should convey the message in a supportive way to avoid panic and
overreaction. A 2003 *New York Times* article by Lawrence Altman
concluded, "Many doctors and the drug industry promoted use of
hormone therapy a few years ago despite the lack of evidence from
clinical trials. But now experts say that experience has taught doctors and society a lesson in the need to exert extreme caution in in-
troducing new therapies."

Alone or combined with progestin, estrogen is not recommended
for women who meet the descriptions in the serious risk list below,
and it may not be safe for women with any of the characteristics in
the relative risk list.

Serious Risk

- Stroke
- Recent heart attack
- Breast cancer (including family history)
- Uterine cancer
- Acute liver disease
- Ovarian cancer
- Gallbladder disease
- Pancreatic disease
- Recent blood clot
- Undiagnosed vaginal bleeding

Relative Risk

- Cigarette smoking
- High blood pressure
- Benign breast disease
- Benign uterine disease
- Endometriosis
- Pancreatitis
- Epilepsy
- Migraine headaches

Subjective Complaints (These are symptoms you may have if you decide to take hormones.)

- Nausea
- Headaches
- Breakthrough bleeding
- Depression
- Fluid retention
- Dry eye syndrome

■ Natural Progesterone

Some recent research suggests that replacing progesterone may be more important than replacing estrogen. Dr. Joel Hargrove of Vanderbilt University has shown very good clinical results using an average starting does of 0.5 mg estradiol and 100 mg natural progesterone in a single capsule daily. Dr. Hargrove's studies show an improvement in vaginal dryness, hot flashes, and bone health.

According to Dr. Christiane Northrup, former president of the American Holistic Medical Association, natural progesterone is free of side effects and is different from synthetic progestins such as Provera. Five mg of Provera is equal to 100 mg of natural progesterone. Dr. Northrup suggests using formulations such as Progest or Bio Balance, although she does acknowledge that Provera may be needed in cases of heavy bleeding.

A safe way to replace progesterone is to use a natural progesterone cream. This can provide relief of menopausal symptoms while stimulating your body's production and regulation of estrogen and other hormones. Skin preparations (transdermal form) of progesterone creams can be used to counterbalance estrogen in women with an intact uterus as long as the endometrium is monitored. A physician performs an endometrial biopsy when there is postmenopausal bleeding. Ideally hormone levels will be monitored by a physician, although progesterone-containing creams are available over the counter and many women use them.

Dr. Northrup cautions that most concoctions sold as yam creams contain little or no progesterone. These include Progestone 10 and Progestone-HP and Yamcon. Although, the active ingredient in yams is used to manufacture progesterone, there are insufficient data to indicate that a yam cream will help you in the same manner as a natural progesterone in standardized amounts. The usual dose of creams that contain 400 mg/ounce is one-quarter to one-third teaspoon on the skin one to two times per day. There is no danger of overdose, and some women use an entire tube or jar a week with no ill effects.

Other experts disagree. They say wild yam, the staple food in several tropical countries, is a good source of a steroid used in the manufacture of the pill and other sex hormone preparations. In 1970, the Mexican government nationalized the yam industry as a safeguard. This pushed up prices and the drug companies looked elsewhere for a cheap source. In China, where doctors regard Western corticosteroids as too expensive, several species of yam are used.

■ Bioidentical Hormones

Bioidentical hormones are manufactured to have the same molecular structure as the hormones made by your own body. By contrast, synthetic hormones are intentionally different. Drug companies can't patent a bioidentical structure, so they invent synthetic hormones that can be patented.

Although bioidentical hormones have been around for years, most practitioners are unfamiliar with them. There are several branded versions now available. The dosage regime is generally one-size-fits-all.

If you select this route, talk with your health care practitioner about an individualized approach. Using your hormone panel, your health care practitioner can prescribe a precise dosage of bioidentical estrogens, testosterone, or DHEA (a precursor of the hormone testosterone) that is made up at a compounding pharmacy. You will need to be monitored carefully (a hormone panel every 3 months) to ensure you get symptom relief at the lowest possible dosage. Once balance is restored, you'll need a panel once a year at the time of your annual exam.

I've had women send me e-mails asking, "Are bioidentical hormones better than synthetic hormones?"

They may be better, but they're not perfect. The great appeal of bioidentical hormones is that they are natural and your body can metabolize them as it was designed to do, minimizing side effects. Synthetic hormones are quite strong and often produce intolerable side effects. Also, compounded bioidentical hormones can be matched individually to your needs—something that's impossible with mass-produced products you buy off the shelf.

Dolores, a 39-year-old woman who had hot flashes and night sweats, wanted to take bioidentical hormones because she had heard about the European medical studies that suggest they are safer than synthetics. She asked for my opinion.

I told her that it had to be her decision, but European medical studies have suggested that bioidentical hormones are safer than synthetic ones. But caution is advised because they haven't been well studied, especially for long-term use. Never think of any drug as completely safe.

Most women can rebalance their hormones without the use of drugs. The nurse practitioners at a private practice called Women to Women have found that about 85% can find relief through an approach that combines medical-grade nutritional supplements, over-the-counter bioidentical progesterone, and dietary and lifestyle changes. They recommend that every woman start with this combination approach as a foundation of health. For sure, they don't recommend that any hormones be used long term unless essential for symptom relief, and then only with a complete risk assessment. They also don't support the idea that bioidentical hormones should be used indefinitely as some kind of fountain of youth.

■ Deciding Whether to Take Hormones

Prior to taking hormones, you may want to find out whether you are estrogen dominant. This means you already have an excess of estrogen or are progesterone deficient. While estrogen levels will decrease during menopause, they do not fall appreciably until after a woman's last period. In fact, far more women suffer from the effects of estrogen dominance during the transition. And some women can suffer from estrogen dominance for 10 to 15 years, beginning as early as age 35.

All of these signs are exacerbated by stress of all kinds. You may experience moderate to severe symptoms of estrogen dominance as you approach perimenopause. Check which ones you have now or have had. If you have five or more signs or two or more * signs, then estrogen dominance may be causing them. (For information on nutritional approaches to estrogen dominance, see chapter 4.)

- ❑ *breast swelling/tenderness
- ❑ high blood pressure
- ❑ *endometrial cancer
- ❑ *D&C
- ❑ *PMS
- ❑ *menopausal symptoms
- ❑ craving sweets
- ❑ facial pigmentation
- ❑ bruise easily
- ❑ mistiness of vision
- ❑ increased weight around abdomen/hips
- ❑ *difficulty losing weight
- ❑ *gallbladder symptoms
- ❑ *breast cancer
- ❑ endometrial hyperplasia
- ❑ cyclic acne
- ❑ toxemia of pregnancy
- ❑ cramping at ovulation
- ❑ *depression/irritability
- ❑ accident prone
- ❑ flashes of light
- ❑ dark circles under eyes
- ❑ inability to concentrate

- ❑ asthma
- ❑ *fibromyalgia
- ❑ breast fibrocysts/tumors
- ❑ varicose veins
- ❑ backache
- ❑ *heavy or irregular periods
- ❑ infertility
- ❑ *water retention/edema
- ❑ migraines, headaches
- ❑ joint and muscle pain
- ❑ stroke
- ❑ insomnia
- ❑ hemorrhoids, constipation
- ❑ hypoglycemia
- ❑ *hysterectomy

If you decide to take hormones, take the ones that most match those that occur naturally in your body such as progesterone. Natural preparations are preferable to conjugated combinations such as Premarin, which comes from horse's urine. Although superior preparations employing natural hormones are now available, for historical and economic reasons, Premarin continues to be prescribed and is the estrogen employed in most major studies including the Women's Health Initiative.

Regardless of your position on the treatment of pregnant mares, from whose urine this estrogen is extracted, the important point is that Premarin is not a steroid native to the human body. There is some evidence that when Premarin breaks down, it has independent metabolic consequences that aren't understood. Because of concerns about breast cancer being associated with ERT, the use of synthetic hormones incompatible with the human body could be the equivalent of a vast experiment on the human female population.

Dr. Christianne Northrup says that prescriptions for hormones should be tailored to individual needs and varied over the 13 years of the climacteric. If you decide to take HRT, Dr. Northrup suggests a follow-up saliva test in 3 months and a readjustment in dosage then and annually.

Dr. Susan Love's Web site proclaims, "I believe it is okay for women to take HRT for 3 to 5 years for symptom relief during menopause . . . start tapering off over a 6–9 month period or start taking the lowest dose of Premarin (0.3 or 0.15 mg) that you can."

Dr. Steven R. Goldstein, professor of obstetrics and gynecology at the New York Medical Center in Manhattan, states,

> *Every woman should reevaluate exactly why she is on HRT to see whether the benefits outweigh the risks. . . . Hot flashes, sleeplessness and vaginal dryness prevent some women from carrying on day-to-day functions . . . the actual risk of cardiovascular problems and breast cancer vary depending upon the individual's lifestyle and family medical history. . . . Consider the case of a 56-year-old menopausal woman who goes to her doctor complaining of hot flashes. If she is overweight, a smoker, and doesn't exercise, I might suggest she invest in a personal fan.*

The Society for Women's Health Research reminds us that "hot flashes and the like generally subside a few years after a woman enters menopause." Weigh the discomfort of hot flashes, vaginal dryness, and sweating against the possible dangers of heart attack, stroke, blood clots, and breast cancer, knowing that there are natural treatments available that can tone these symptoms down (see chapters 4–9).

Knowing what you do and remembering that medical science is a work in progress, answer the questions that follow and see if hormone replacement is right for you.

1. Hot flashes and sweating ❑ True   ❑ False
   prevent me from functioning.

2. I am at the weight I was   ❑ True   ❑ False
   in high school.

3. I avoid smokers, smoky places,   ❑ True   ❑ False
   and smoking.

4. I exercise for at least   ❑ True   ❑ False
   20 minutes every day.

5. My family has no history of   ❑ True   ❑ False
   breast cancer, stroke, blood clots,
   or heart disease.

Being overweight is a risk factor for heart and circulatory diseases and breast cancer; so are a history of these conditions, not exercising, and smoking. If you have none of these risk factors and are incapacitated by hot flashes and sweating, you might want to consider taking hormone replacement therapy. But even if you answered "True" to all five items, consider that there are also safe natural alternatives to taking hormones.

If you decide to use HRT, use it at the lowest dose that helps and for the shortest time needed. Ask your health care practitioner about using it every other day. For more information on the Women's Health Initiative study results and on the risks and benefits of HRT, go to http://www.nhibi.nih.gov/health/women/index.htm.

■ Surgical Menopause

Olivia was 30 when her physician told her that she should have surgery for fibroids. Her bleeding was heavy and Olivia worried about it, but she'd never had surgery before. She called me, hoping to discuss the pros and cons. She asked, "Should I have a hysterectomy?"

I told her that she needed to discuss this with her physician. There are conditions for which hysterectomy is advisable or medically necessary. They may include ovarian, uterine, or cervical cancer, uncontrollable bleeding, severe endometriosis (lining of the uterus grows in other areas of the pelvis, or adenomyosis (glands inside the uterus grows into the wall of the organ), and abnormal increases in uterine cells, to name a few.

She told me she had fibroids and endometriosis. I told her she should undergo an endometrial biopsy. This kind of biopsy is indicated in any woman over 40 years of age who has longstanding bleeding abnormalities, who is at increased risk for endometrial cancer because of obesity and/or bleeding without ovulation, or who is postmenopausal and whose endometrium is >5 mm on pelvic ultrasound.

A large percentage of hysterectomies are performed to relieve fibroids, endometriosis, or other conditions related to hormonal imbalance. Hysterectomy in these cases may be unnecessary. You may be unaware of alternatives. One thing to remember is that fibroids usually resolve themselves after menopause.

A study of 500 hysterectomies in California found that they were recommended without following medical guidelines 70% of the time, primarily because of incomplete diagnostic evaluations or failure to try conservative treatments. For example, 45% of women with abnormal uterine bleeding didn't have an endometrial biopsy before surgery, 21% of women with pain or bleeding didn't receive a trial of medical treatment first, and 14% of women had characteristics that made them inappropriate candidates for hysterectomy.

Another study of 700 nonemergency hysterectomies performed at seven health maintenance organizations (HMOs) and reviewed by a panel of medical experts determined that 16% of these surgeries were "inappropriate" and another 25% were of questionable benefit. A common inappropriate reason for hysterectomy was reoccurrence of noncancerous fibroid tumors of less than 12 weeks duration, associated with mild bleeding but without any discomfort.

From 1991 to 1999, the HERS Foundation received reports of harmful effects and adverse outcomes from 621 women who responded to a questionnaire. (It's not clear why HERS obtained opposite results from the Scott and White Clinic study reported on page 23 of this book, but they could have used a different population or asked different questions.) Some of the negative effects HERS found after hysterectomy included:

- Personality changes, loss of energy, irritability, and profound fatigue in more than 75% of respondents
- Loss of sexual desire and inability to return to previous activities in more than 70% of respondents
- Loss of stamina, difficulty socializing, loss of short-term memory, loss of pleasure in intercourse, loss of sexuality and sensuality, less frequent intercourse, and loss of pleasure in foreplay in more than 60% of respondents
- Back pain, hot flashes, anxiety, stiffness, suicidal thoughts, loss of sensation in vagina, muscle aches, insomnia, loss of orgasm, bone and joint pain, loss of lubrication, and loss of sexual organ sensation in more than 50% of respondents

The percentages of negative reactions to hysterectomy were remarkably similar whether the women had a simple hysterectomy (removal of only the uterus) or had one or both ovaries removed. In the HERS study, 97.7% of the women were given little or no prior information about the acknowledged adverse effects of hysterectomy, although this information is a legal requisite of consent for treatment. Nora W. Coffey, president of HERS, makes the point, "Doctors often frighten women into consenting and give them false and misleading information." HERS provides information about specific alternatives to hysterectomy, free information by mail, telephone counseling, CDs and audio and videotapes, physician referrals for treatment, a free lending library, and more. For details, go to http://www.hersfoundation.com or call toll-free at (888)750-4377.

Always weigh the consequences of a hysterectomy prior to deciding. The loss of hormonal balance can create myriad symptoms including premature aging, weight gain, loss of immune function, and more. There are also other complications such as heightened incidence of yeast infections and urinary incontinence. The estrogen made by the ovaries plays a protective role in your health, so a complete hysterectomy prior to menopause increases the risk of heart disease and other problems. The testosterone made by the ovaries (yes, women have testosterone, too, just as men have estrogen) plays an important role in sexual desire and response, so after an oophorectomy (loss of both ovaries) you could suffer a loss of libido and sexual enjoyment.

If you enter menopause as a result of hysterectomy, you could face years of taking hormones to restore your hormonal balance. The synthetic hormones commonly used in HRT have been shown to have significant health risks (see the information earlier in this chapter about hormones), so many women use bioidentical hormones.

Your level of estrogen before surgery may predict your post-surgery experience. The higher the level of estrogen you have, the more daunting your experience can be after surgery. How do you know what your level of estrogen is? If you're full-figured, the odds are you have high estrogen levels. You can also get a hormone panel from your physician as part of your decision-making process. The results can serve as a baseline to help restore hormone balance after surgery. HERS advises:

> *"Take charge of your body and don't allow your vital organs to be removed needlessly. Both your uterus and ovaries have complex and important functions in your body long after your childbearing years are over."*

Take your time. An elective hysterectomy means you have time to consider carefully the pros and cons and to prepare properly for surgery so you can reduce your chances of complications.

Consider trying a holistic program (see chapter 4–9 for ideas) as a natural alternative to hysterectomy. If that approach doesn't relieve symptoms, you can always choose to go forward with the surgery.

> *Darla, a 36-year-old woman, had been overweight her entire life. She had a high estrogen level and suffered from pain and vaginal bleeding. After weighing the pros and cons of hysterectomy and evaluating the heavy bleeding and discomfort she endured, she decided to have surgery. She asked, "How so I prepare so that I can get through this operation?"*

I told her about a great book called *Prepare for Surgery, Heal Faster: A Guide of Mind-Body Techniques* by Peggy Huddleston, with a foreword by Christianne Northrup. There is an audiotape version designed to be listened to during surgery.

Darla decided to use a bioidentical low-dose progesterone cream and developed a holistic program (using the information in this book) to help prepare for the hormonal changes ahead. Once Darla had her surgery, she gave me a call and we focused on her next question: "How do I recover now that I don't have a uterus or ovaries?"

I had already told her that complete hysterectomy triggers a medical menopause. To ease this transition, many women will be advised to use estrogen right after surgery short term, then wean off in a few months. Marcelle Pick, OB/Gyn nurse practitioner, and Marcy Holmes, nurse practitioner and certified menopause clinician for Women to Women, recommend a bioidentical estradiol patch and low-dose progesterone cream combined with natural nondrug approaches.

One of the participants in my menopause study, a 69-year-old woman, underwent a complete hysterectomy in the 1970s. She did not share anything about the reason for surgery other than that she had premenopausal depression in 1976 and used an Estraderm patch after surgery. "The patch helped my muscle pain and spasms," she told me, convinced it also helped with "my depression, which was due to a chemical imbalance."

Keep in mind that all forms of hormone medication after hysterectomy are optional, and you may choose to wait to see how you feel. There's no rush to start hormones. If you've had a complete hysterectomy at a young age, many practitioners recommend estrogen supplementation until you are 45 to 50, when estrogen would normally begin to decline. (There is no exact time to stop; it depends on how you're doing.) Since your uterus has been removed, you do not need prescription-strength progesterone to offset the estrogen. Marcelle Pick and Marcy Holmes recommend using a low-dose progesterone cream instead. Remember that estrogen and progesterone should always be in balance together.

The removal of the ovaries doubles the odds of suffering low testosterone with its adverse effects on libido and sexual enjoyment. Some women adapt and make testosterone in other areas of the body, such as the adrenal glands, but this adaptation can take time.

■ Medical Information

One of the participants in my menopause study, a 45-year-old woman, said,

> If I had had the choice, I would love to have had a child, but I had an emergency hysterectomy 7 years ago which included removal of the ovaries. I had a female OB/GYN who had no compassion whatsoever. As a pediatric nurse, I had essentially no experience or background with menopause. The skin changes really concerned me as everything was so exaggerated. No matter what I asked her, she just answered with "You're taking your Premarin, aren't you?" So 5 years ago I decided I wasn't going to be demeaned by her anymore, so I haven't been to a GYN since. I get my annual and bum prescriptions for Premarin from various health care providers at work.

While you're making decisions about your menopause process, it's important to find a compassionate physician or nurse practitioner and keep that person updated. Consumers have been complaining for years about the lack of physician–patient communication, and you may have experienced some difficulties yourself.

The Internet has just upped the complaint. A digital divide between patients and physicians is creeping into many medical offices, says Dr. Roe A. Roberts of Midwestern State University, Wichita Falls, Texas. She has been studying the effects of encouraging patients to be informed and educated. In the 1980s, this tactic was viewed as a way of improving care and controlling costs through a physician-driven approach that provided select information to patients and training to perform select technical activities. Today, self-management or self-care involves a less physician-controlled approach driven by consumer access to the Internet. Doctors who aren't open to this more active role for consumers and who try to keep a tight rein on information and activities may find themselves left out in the cold, according to Dr. Roberts.

She drew these conclusions after reviewing the studies on patient uses of the Internet and of discussion lists available on the Internet dealing with health-related topics. Consumers who used the Internet tended to be more educated and have higher incomes. They also used the Internet primarily to search for medical information. A majority of patients declared that the information they found was better than the information given to them by their doctors.

About 60% of consumers who surf the Internet for health-related information don't discuss what they find with their physicians, but 24% use the information for self-care. It's wise to discuss your self-care actions with your health care provider just to make sure that whatever you're doing works well with your medical treatment. Be sure to find someone you can work with and feel good about.

Unfortunately, many physicians respond negatively to consumers who approach them with health information obtained from the Internet. The reason for this may have more to do with your physician than with you. Dr. Roberts believes physician reactions are due to a lack of knowledge on their part. She says that a study in 2002 found that consumers are more computer literate than their physicians, more able to use Internet search engines to answer specific medical questions, have better Internet access, and are better able to find new treatments and research. Dr. Roberts says, "One of the chief things I'm seeing is that doctors are telling patients, 'Don't go to the Internet. Don't talk online about health matters.'"

Dr. Roberts says consumers need to be able to discuss the information they gather in an open, nonjudgmental environment. What physicians may not understand is that there is research to back the positive effects of surfing the Net. According to one study, consumers who self-managed their health by gathering information, formulating action plans, and carrying them out reduced their hospitalizations, physician visits, and lost workdays. That alone ought to be enough to convince any health care practitioner of the benefits of consumer involvement in their care.

Some information on the Web may not be valid. You can find abstracts of research articles at www.pubmed.com and complete articles in medical journals at your local hospital library. Both provide the most valid information available. Even then, check to see who supported the research. Drug companies often fund studies and buy ads. This leads to the publication of primarily drug-based studies, so the findings can be biased. Your reference librarian can also help you find appropriate sources of information.

Don't let a physician's reluctance to discuss your questions and information deter you from learning all you can about your menopause. If your physician isn't open to discussing your questions and comments, consider finding another health care provider. Whatever you do, keep up with the research about menopause because new self-care measures are being found all the time. As you read the studies, be sure to take into account the following factors: the type of sample (mice or rat or petri dish results may or may not be applicable to humans), the size of the sample (a small sample usually indicates less evidence in support of the findings), whether a control group was used (a control group provides evidence that a novel effect didn't create the findings), whether the researchers and those providing treatment were blinded to who received the treatment under study (a double-blind, placebo trial is best), who funded the study, and who collected the data (pressure to find the results wanted by the funding group or lead researcher can sway results).

This chapter has provided a great deal of medical information. Take your time and digest what is relevant for you. Once you've done that, use the suggested resources to learn more. Remember that you know your body better than anyone else. Find a health care practitioner who will work with you and support you and your unique needs. You deserve it.

PART II

Holistic Approaches

Nutrition

At age 30, Harriet had breast cancer and a double mastectomy. After that, her husband refused to have sex with her, even after she'd had breast reconstruction. Their marriage broke up, and she felt terrible about herself. Harriet had started to binge eat at night, eating half a gallon of ice milk or half a pie on some evenings. When she started to have menopausal changes at age 45, she turned to nutrition to help her because she couldn't take hormones. She joined one of my nutrition groups and started to learn about the foods that could help relieve hot flashes, insomnia, and bleeding. As she learned more and more about what she'd been putting into her body and the kinds of foods that could be beneficial, she started to lose weight and thrive.

Her story bears out the old saying, "You are what you eat!" Research findings also provide evidence that food is a very important medicine.

Unfortunately, the typical American high-fat, high-protein, high-sugar diet is associated with:

- Increased risk of breast, ovarian, bowel, kidney, and uterine cancer
- Increased risk of cardiovascular disease
- Increased risk of varicose veins
- Increased risk of gallstones
- Constipation
- Heavy menstrual bleeding
- Increased risk of osteoporosis
- Increased endometriosis symptoms
- Excess body fat

You can reduce menopause changes and risks just by eating different foods. This chapter provides evidence-based (and 99.99% of the time, research-based) findings that support the use of specific foods that can help you have a better postmenopause.

This chapter, and the remaining chapters 5 through 9, are organized alphabetically by menopause change or risk including breast cancer, cold hands, depression, fatigue, hair loss/thinning, headaches, heart disease, hot flashes, insomnia/sleep problems, itching, joint and muscle pain, memory loss, menstrual bleeding, fuzzy thinking, osteoporosis, sex drive/intercourse discomfort, dry/scaly skin, urinary symptoms, and weight gain. You can also look up menopause changes in the index at the back of the book.

■ Breast Cancer and Other Cancers

Avoid:

Meat and Other Animal Products Many animals are treated with hormones to hasten growth. Meat also contains saturated fat. Avoid all dairy products except for unsweetened low-fat yogurt.

Junk Foods Processed refined food, saturated fats, salt, sugar, and white flour are non-nourishing to the body. This means pies, cakes, cookies, doughnuts, many muffins and cereals, candy, and other desserts and sweets.

Supplements Containing Iron Iron may be used by tumors to promote their growth.

Focus On

Apples Consumption of fruits and vegetables has been associated with a low incidence of cancers. Several studies have shown that fresh apples inhibit tumor cell growth and production of new cancer cells.

Calcium-Rich Foods Calcium may help prevent cancer. Calcium comes in many forms, some more adsorbable than others. Probably the most absorbable form comes from eating a diet that includes daily amounts of one or more of the following foods:

almonds	dulse (seaweed)	parsley
asparagus	fennel	peppermint
blackstrap molasses	figs	prunes
broccoli	filberts	salmon with bones
buttermilk	flaxseeds	sardines
cabbage	goat's milk	seafood
carob	green leafy vegetables	sesame seeds
cheese (soy)	kale	tofu
chickory	kelp	turnip greens
collards	mustard greens	watercress
dandelion greens	oats	

Just because you eat calcium-rich foods or take calcium supplements doesn't mean you are getting enough calcium. Factors that affect calcium absorption include:

- A diet high in protein, fat, and or sugar reduces calcium uptake.
- A diet high in oxalic acid (almonds, beet greens, cashews, Swiss chard, cocoa/chocolate, kale, rhubarb, soybeans and cooked spinach) interferes with calcium absorption.

- Consuming meat, refined grains, alcoholic beverages, junk foods, coffee, soft drinks, excess salt, white flour products, and soft drinks leads to loss of calcium from the body.
- The amino acid lysine is necessary for calcium absorption. Food sources of lysine include eggs, fish, lima beans, potatoes, and soy products.
- Heavy exercise hinders calcium uptake, but moderate exercise promotes it.
- A diet based on vegetables, fruits, and whole grains that contain significant amounts of calcium and magnesium and low levels of phosphorus is a good meal plan.

Calcium Supplements

• Take calcium supplements in small doses spread throughout the day and before bedtime for best absorption. Your last dose of the day can promote sound sleep.

• Avoid supplements containing D1-calcium-phosphate. It's insoluble and interferes with the absorption of nutrients in a multivitamin or multimineral.

• Avoid taking antacids as a source of calcium. When taken in sufficient quantity to serve as a major source of calcium, they neutralize stomach acid needed for calcium absorption.

• Avoid calcium supplements if you have a history of kidney stones or kidney disease.

• Check your supplement. Calcium in the form of calcium carbonate is only absorbable when taken with a meal, and even then it's the most poorly absorbed (only 5%–10%). Unlike the other inorganic forms of the mineral, calcium carbonate requires (and binds) the most acid. More acid is then required for the digestion of proteins or else malabsorption (and indigestion) can occur.

• Choose one of the organic forms. Absorption can run anywhere from 25% to as high as 95%. The best absorbed of the commercially available types are calcium orotate (90%–95% absorbed), closely followed by calcium aspartate (85% absorbed). But they are not only the most expensive; they're also the hardest to find. Another really good one is calcium ascorbate, which gives you the benefit of vitamin C. The next best are the amino acid chelates, 65% to 80% absorption, but these are still fairly expensive and not as easily found. The best compromise of price, percentage of elemental calcium, and absorption is calcium citrate. The absorption is 30% to 35%, and the citric acid reduces the amount of stomach acids required for absorption.

Don't take calcium as a supplement by itself. Calcium is not found in nature (in edible form) without magnesium, and they should always be taken together. Studies show that calcium alone may even be preferentially laid down in arterial walls rather than in bones. Phosphorous is also needed with calcium, but most people get enough of that mineral. For healthy bones, the calcium must have not only magnesium but manganese, silica, boron, strontium, vitamin D in high doses, vitamin C, vitamin B12, and more, which is why taking a daily multivitamin or eating to ensure you ingest these other nutrients is also important. Fortunately, most calcium supplements aren't expensive, so you can take a lot of one that your body doesn't absorb well and do okay, as long as you're getting a multimineral supplement that has the other needed minerals in it.

According to Dr. David McCarron, a nephrologist at Oregon Health Sciences University in Portland, calcium binds to fatty acids and neutralizes them, restricting their tendency to encourage cells to multiply out of control and develop into tumors. An article in *US News and World Report* says that on average American consumers take 30% less than the 1,000 mg (1,500 mg for postmenopausal women) recommended daily.

Magnesium is available in dried pumpkin seeds (two handfuls a day contain nearly all of the 320 milligrams needed by women). Magnesium is also abundant in nuts, legumes, rice bran, whole-grain cereals and breads, soy, wheat germ, figs, green leafy vegetables (chickory, collards, dandelion greens, mustard greens, parsley, turnip greens, spinach, and kale). Eat the last two raw so oxalic acid doesn't interfere with absorption.

Find potassium in raw spinach, cabbage, cauliflower, tomatoes, carrots, soy, wheat germ, and eggs. Find vitamin D in eggs, salmon, tuna, sardines, sweet potatoes, alfalfa sprouts, and parsley. If you have a lawn, you probably have dandelions. If you don't use pesticides or herbicides on your grass or spill gasoline while mowing, it may be safe to eat the stems. Dandelion greens are a rich source of vitamin D, not to mention a strong liver cleanser. Exposing the face and arms to the sun for 15 minutes three times a week is an effective way to ensure adequate amounts of vitamin D in your body.

Carotenoids Damage to DNA, the principal carrier of genetic information, may be important to the development of most cancers. Some of this damage is caused by free radicals, which can be inactivated by beta-carotene, alpha-carotene, lycopene, lutein, and other carotenoids and antioxidants. One study showed that after drinking a daily serving of tomato juice, carrot juice, or a spinach-containing beverage for 2 weeks, damage to DNA was reduced.

Iron Iron is an important nutrient associated with bone health. Collagen, an integral component of bone, cannot be produced without it. A recent study of menopausal women found that those who consumed 18 mg iron a day, along with adequate calcium (1,500 mg a day), had the greatest bone mineral density. But the average American diet contains about 6 mg iron for every 1,000 calories. Most women average only 9 to 10 mg iron daily, or as little as half their daily recommendation, which is why it's important to watch what you eat.

Caffeine, fiber-rich foods, and calcium supplements can reduce iron absorption. If you take iron in a supplement, take it separately from calcium or calcium-rich foods. Vitamin C slightly increases iron absorption. Taking vitamin A with iron helps treat iron deficiency, since vitamin A helps the body use iron stored in the liver.

Since heme iron from meat is associated with heart disease and iron supplements are not well absorbed, your best bet might be to obtain sufficient iron from nonheme iron sources. Combine the following foods to obtain 18 mg iron every day:

1 cup soy flour = 8.8 mg

1 cup wheat germ = 5.5 mg

⅓ cup sesame seeds = 5.2 mg

¼ cup Brewer's yeast = 5 milligrams

2 tablespoons blackstrap (unrefined) molasses = 4.6 mg

1 cup brown rice = 4 mg

⅓ cup sunflower seeds = 3.5 mg

½ cup almonds = 3.3 mg

½ cup unsalted cashews = 2.9 mg

1 cup bean soup = 2.8 mg

1 cup macaroni and cheese = 2.6 mg

1 cup spaghetti with tomatoes and cheese = 2 mg

½ cup baked beans = 2 mg

1 cup yellow cornmeal = 1.8 mg

10 dried apricots = 1.7 mg

1 cup oatmeal = 1.7 mg

10 dates = 1.6 mg

½ cup raw English walnuts = 1.5 mg

1 cup split pea soup = 1.4 mg

2 slices whole-wheat bread = 1.4 mg

4 buckwheat or whole-wheat pancakes (4 in.) = 1.3 mg

3 oz. turkey = 1.2 mg

1 raw stalk broccoli = 1.1 mg

3 oz. tuna in water = 1 mg

¼ cup raisins = 1 mg

If you don't eat enough of these foods, cook in iron pots and pans to obtain your iron.

Grapes Grapes contain *resveratrol,* a natural phytoalexin with anticancer activity. This substance has the ability to kill cancer cells.

Low-Fat and High-Fiber Diet Breast cancer risk increases after menopause, especially if you're taking hormones. In a study of 89,602 postmenopausal women, researchers found that high-fiber and low-fat intakes were associated with a lower risk of post-menopausal breast cancer. High-fiber foods include apples, bananas, pears, dried figs, dried prunes, raw strawberries, kidney beans, cooked split peas, raisin bran, shredded wheat, and cooked lentils. Two to three servings of fruits and three to five servings of vegetables every day should meet your fiber requirements of 20–30 grams. A fiber content chart for common foods can be found at www.slrbc.org/heathinfo under dietary fiber.

"To get the most bang for your buck in protecting against serious diseases, eat 'powerhouse' fruits and vegetables packed with the most nutrients and antioxidants," says Marilyn S. Nanney of the St. Louis University School of Public Health in the March 2004 issue of the *Journal of the American Dietetic Association.* Still in doubt about which fruits and vegetables to eat? Choose the darker colored ones over the lighter ones. Carrots, winter squash, cantaloupe, and oranges, top corn, and cauliflower is better than onion. Tomatoes, red peppers, and strawberries are more potent than apples in most cases. Broccoli and spinach provide more benefits than iceberg lettuce or celery.

Lettuce, Onions, and Red Wine According to the International Agency for Research on Cancer, lettuce, onions, and red wine are important sources of dietary *flavonoids* (crystalline substances found in plants) that are probably responsible for protecting the body against carcinogens. (Since alcohol can enhance hot flashes, get the same benefits by eating grapes.)

Maitake Mushrooms Maitake mushrooms, an edible fungi you can find in your grocery store, inhibits tumor formation from environmental toxins and primes the body to release immune enhancers including beta glucans, helper T cells, and natural killer cells. Experiments suggest that maitake inhibits metastasis (the spread of cancer) and causes cancer cell death for long-term cancer suppression. One study found that 68.8% of breast cancers regressed or there was significant symptom improvement. Animal studies have supported the use of maitake mushrooms for long-term cancer suppression.

Mandarin Oranges and Other Citrus Fruits   Mandarin oranges and other citrus fruits contain *limonoids* that have been shown to significantly inhibit the growth of estrogen receptor (negative and positive) human breast cancer cells in culture. These limonoids are also capable of killing breast cancer cells.

Soy and Soy Products   Several types of studies show the protective effects of soy against breast cancer. In laboratory study in which human breast cancer cells were mixed with high amounts of *isoflavones, biochanin A, daidzein,* and *genistein* (all found in soy products), the growth of cancerous cells was stunted by as much as 30%.

In another study, women who ate 60 grams of soy protein a day for 1 month showed a lengthened follicular phase by an average of 2.5 days. A longer follicular phase is associated with a reduction in estrogen's negative effects on breast tissue, indicating a possible mechanism for why soy has an anti–breast cancer effect.

A study published in *Cancer Epidemiological Biomarkers and Prevention* provided evidence that soy foods prevent breast cancer. Another study published in the *International Journal of Cancer* found that a combination of soy phytochemical concentrate and green tea inhibited tumor growth. The researchers concluded that dietary soy plus green tea showed potential for inhibiting progression of estrogen-dependent breast cancer.

Although there is no relevant clinical research to show the opposite, many physicians consider soy contraindicated in women who have estrogen receptor–positive tumors. The only available research (which does not appear to be equivalent to human studies or even to healthy mice or mice with breast cancer) was completed on mice who had had their ovaries and thymuses removed and were implanted with human breast cancer cells; these mice were then given genistein, a phytochemical found in soy products. Isolating genistein this way and using a sample so unlike postmenopausal women does not provide strong evidence to support the idea that soy contributes to human breast cancer.

Raspberries Black raspberries have been shown to inhibit the development of chemically induced cancers in rodents.

Strawberries Strawberries contain *isothiocyanates* that have been shown to inhibit tumor growth. One cancer-preventive agent in the berries is ellagic acid, but there are other inhibitors. Strawberries that are grown with composted soil are more potent inhibitors of cancer.

■ Cold Hands

Cold hands can be a symptom of *hypothyroidism,* a condition caused by an underproduction of thyroid hormone. Symptoms include fatigue, loss of appetite, inability to tolerate cold, a slow heart rate, weight gain, painful premenstrual periods, a milky discharge from the breasts, fertility problems, muscle weakness, muscle cramps, dry and scaly skin, a yellow-orange coloration in the skin, yellow bumps on the eyelids, hair loss, recurrent infections, constipation, depression, difficulty concentrating, slow speech, goiter and drooping, swollen eyes.

Avoid:

Foods and Supplements That Suppress Thyroid Function Brussels sprouts, peaches, pears, spinach, turnips, cabbage, broccoli, kale and mustard greens, white bread, sugary cereals, and any foods containing any form of sugar may further suppress thyroid function. Avoid taking more than 500 milligrams of vitamin C at once. Get your vitamin C from strawberries, peppers, cauliflower, parsley, watercress, onions, and alfalfa sprouts. Avoid taking more than 400 I.U. of vitamin E daily. Avoid drinking water that contains fluoride or chlorine. They block iodine receptors in the thyroid gland. Avoid using fluoride toothpaste.

Focus On:

Kelp Put it on your salads and in your soups, casseroles, and so forth. Kelp contains iodine, the basic substance of thyroid hormone.

Vitamin B-Complex–Rich Foods The B-vitamins improve cellular oxygenation and energy that is needed for proper digestion, immune function, and thyroid function. Your daily intake should include blackstrap molasses, egg yolks, parsley, apricots, dates, prunes, fish or chicken, sunflower seeds, oats, green peas, lima beans, wheat germ, grapes, mushrooms, cauliflower, and filberts or peanuts.

Vitamin E–Rich Foods Foods include wheat germ, peanuts, asparagus, oats, eggs, and sweet potatoes. Drink distilled water only.

■ Depression, Nervousness, and Irritability

Avoid:

Wheat Products Wheat gluten has been linked to depressive disorders.

Artificial Sweeteners Artificial sweeteners such as Equal and NutraSweet contain the amino acid phenylalanine that can be highly allergic to depressed people.

Sugar The body reacts more quickly to sugar than to complex carbohydrates (fruits, vegetables, and whole grains), releasing quick energy that is quickly followed by fatigue and depression.

Foods High in Saturated Fats Meat and frieds foods, such as hamburgers and French fries interfere with blood flow by blocking arteries and small blood vessels and causing blood cells to clump together, resulting in poor circulation, especially in the brain, sluggishness, slow thinking, and fatigue.

Alcohol, Caffeine, and Processed Foods Each of these stressors can add to nervousness and irritability.

Focus On:

Biotin Biotin deficiency can lead to depression. To ward off this event, eat more brewer's nutritional yeast (avoid if susceptible to yeast infections), cooked egg yolks, poultry, saltwater fish, soybeans, and whole grains.

Calcium Calcium may help lift depression and relieve nervousness and irritability. Calcium comes in many forms, some more absorbable than others. Probably the most absorbable form comes from eating a diet that includes daily amounts of one or more of the following foods:

almonds	dulse (seaweed)	peppermint
asparagus	fennel	prunes
blackstrap molasses	figs	salmon with bones
broccoli	filberts	sardines
buttermilk	flaxseeds	seafood
cabbage	goat's milk	sesame seeds
carob	kale	tofu
cheese (soy)	kelp	turnip greens
chickory	mustard greens	watercress
collards	oats	
dandelion greens	parsley	

Fish Oil A study reported in *Science News* provided evidence that fish oil helps stabilize the volatile moods that accompany depression. You can either take fish oil capsules (follow directions on label) or eat 3–4 ounces of Artic salmon, Spanish mackerel, herring, or sardines.

Magnesium Magnesium guards against depression, nervousness, and irritability. Magnesium-rich foods include whole-grain bread and cereals, peas, soy, wheat germ, nuts, figs, green leafy vegetables, such as spinach, and kale.

SAMe   S-adenosyl-methione is a popular supplement synthesized from the amino acid (protein builder) methionine and is found throughout the body. In a study reported in the *American Journal of Psychiatry*, by the end of the second week of a small trial, 66% of the SAMe participants had a reduction in depression versus 22% of participants taking imipramine (Tofranil), an antidepressant. SAMe had no side effects, while reactions to imipramine included drowsiness, heart arrhythmias, low or high blood pressure, fatigue, nausea, rash, increased perspiration, headache, changes in blood sugar, sensitivity to light/sun, water retention, jaundice, muscle spasticity and uncontrollable movements, and blood cell disturbances. Imipramine cannot be taken or must be taken with caution by those with glaucoma, psychosis, diabetes, hyperthyroidism, kidney or liver disorders, asthma, epilepsy, heart or blood vessel disease, or urine retention. In sum, SAMe works better and has fewer adverse effects. If you are depressed and on an antidepressant, talk to your health care practitioner about SAMe.

Vitamin B6   Pyridoxine deficiency can lead to depression. Food sources include brewer's nutritional yeast, (avoid if susceptible to yeast infections), carrots, chicken, eggs, fish, peas, spinach, sunflower seeds, walnuts, wheat germ, avocado, bananas, beans, blackstrap molasses, broccoli, brown rice and other whole grains, cabbage, cantaloupe, corn, dulse, plantains, potatoes, soybeans, and tempeh.

Vitamin B12   In one study participants deficient in vitamin B12 were twice as likely to be severely depressed as were participants who had sufficient vitamin B12. Foods to eat to ensure you have a sufficient amount of this vitamin include organically produced liver, clams, oysters, sardines, Spanish mackerel, trout, herring, and eggs. Other vitamin B12 foods you can find at your local health food store are nutritional yeast, sea vegetables (kombu, dulse, and wakame), tempeh, natto, miso, and kelp.

■ Dizziness

Avoid:

Substances Associated with Dizziness Do not consume any fatty fried foods, sugar (in any form), salt, or caffeine.

Focus On:

Iron If you're dizzy, you might be deficient in iron. If you aren't getting enough iron (due to eating insufficient amounts of iron-rich foods or due to heavy bleeding or other causes), make sure you increase your intake of the follow iron-rich foods and be sure to use iron pots for cooking:

almonds	kidney and lima beans	raisins
avocados	lentils	sesame seeds
beets	millet	soybeans
blackstrap molasses	peaches	watercress
dates	pears	whole-grain breads
eggs	prunes	and cereals
green leafy vegetables	pumpkin	

Magnesium Magnesium can help prevent dizziness. Magnesium-rich foods include whole-grain bread and cereals, peas, soy, wheat germ, nuts, figs, green leafy vegetables, spinach, and kale.

Salt Another source of dizziness is low blood pressure. Researchers at John Hopkins University School of Medicine in Baltimore discovered that if your blood pressure is 115/65 or lower and/or you have been diagnosed with chronic fatigue syndrome, salt therapy may help.

Salt makes the body retain water, increasing blood volume. Blood pressure then rises. (This is why individuals with high blood pressure or those with a lifestyle likely to encourage it are told to cut down on salt.) Speak to your health care provider about starting salt therapy if you think your dizziness is due to low blood pressure.

Vitamin B6 Vitamin B6 (pyridoxine) deficiency can lead to dizziness. Food sources include brewer's nutritional yeast (avoid if susceptible to yeast infections), carrots, chicken, eggs, fish, peas, spinach, sunflower seeds, walnuts, wheat germ, avocados, bananas, beans, blackstrap molasses, broccoli, brown rice and other whole grains, cabbage, cantaloupe, corn, dulse, plantains, potatoes, soybeans, and tempeh.

■ Fatigue

Avoid:

Foods That Are Apt to Create Fatigue Milk, sugar, chocolate, eggs, and wheat (including bread, pasta, and cereal) are the foods most likely to create fatigue.

Focus On:

Calcium Calcium may provide energy and reduce fatigue. Calcium comes in many forms, some more absorbable than others. Probably the most absorbable form comes from eating a diet rich in calcium that includes daily amounts of one or more of the following foods:

almonds	cheese (soy)	filberts
asparagus	chickory	flaxseeds
blackstrap molasses	collards	goat's milk
broccoli	dandelion greens	kale
buttermilk	dulse (seaweed)	kelp
cabbage	fennel	mustard greens
carob	figs	oats

parsley	sardines	turnip greens
peppermint	seafood	watercress
prunes	sesame seeds	
salmon with bones	tofu	

Chromium   Need more energy? Research presented at the 63rd Scientific Sessions of the American Diabetes Association in New Orleans in 2004 showed 400 micrograms of chromium combined with 1.8 grams of CLA (conjugated linoleic acid found in soy, safflower, or peanut oil) increased muscle glycogen production by 33%, indicating that carbs are converted more efficiently into energy when the two nutrients are taken together.

Folic Acid   Fatigue can be a sign of folic acid deficiency. To protect against fatigue, eat more barley, brewer's nutritional yeast (avoid if suspectible to yeast infections), brown rice, chicken, dates, green leafy vegetables, legumes, lentils, liver, mushrooms, oranges, split peas, root vegetables, salmon, tuna, wheat germ, whole-grain cereals and breads.

Iron   A major source of fatigue is iron deficiency. A Ball State University study gave premenopausal women either tofu or tofu plus orange juice. They found the iron was more easily absorbed when the tofu (iron source) was supplemented with orange juice containing vitamin C (ascorbic acid). If you plan to use tofu as a major source of iron in your meal plan, make sure you eat it with fruits or vegetables that contain vitamin C, including citrus fruit, strawberries, peppers, broccoli, cauliflower, parsley, watercress, cabbage, onions, sprouts, and raw spinach.

Kelp   This sea vegetable can enhance thyroid function, thereby reducing fatigue. Find it in the seasoning section of health food stores (sprinkle on salads, soups, casseroles, etc.) or in bulk.

Vitamin B6   Pyridoxine deficiency can lead to fatigue. Food sources include brewer's nutritional yeast (avoid if susceptible to yeast infections), carrots, chicken, eggs, fish, peas, spinach, sunflower seeds, walnuts, wheat germ, avocados, bananas, beans, blackstrap molasses, broccoli, brown rice and other whole grains, cabbage, cantaloupe, corn, dulse, plantains, potatoes, soybeans, tempeh, onions, alfalfa sprouts, and raw spinach.

■ Hair Loss/Thinning

It's normal to lose 40–100 hairs a day. More extreme hair loss occurs after having a baby and after menopause. Heredity, hormones, and aging are probably involved in most hair loss, although surgery, radiation exposure, skin disease, sudden weight loss, high fever, iron deficiency, diabetes, thyroid disease, drugs, stress, poor diet, and vitamin deficiencies can play a role, too. The consumption of large amounts of caffeine may cause a shortage of B vitamins in the body.

Good nutrition is a must for beautiful hair. Are you eating 10 fresh organically grown vegetables and fruits a day? If you can manage that, you're well on your way to healthier hair.

Avoid:

Substances That Leach B-Vitamins from the Body B-Vitamins are important to hair health. The consumption of large amounts of caffeine may cause a shortage of B-vitamins in the body. Alcohol and stress have a similar effect.

Focus On:

Biotin Biotin may prevent hair loss. Eat more brown rice, bulgar, green peas, lentils, oats, soy products (soy burgers, soy cheese, soy milk), and walnuts. Sunflower seeds are also good but high in calories. If you don't like the taste, put them in salads or cereal, or you can toast them with a little soy sauce for a tasty snack. A handful is a good amount to take every day. Avoid raw egg—it is a biotin robber and a salmonella infection risk.

Coenzyme Q10 Coenzyme Q10 improves scalp circulation and increases tissue oxidation throughout the body. That's why it's been used successfully to prevent heart and gum conditions.

Copper Copper works with zinc to aid hair growth. Food sources include barley, beans, avocados, almonds, beets, blackstrap molasses, broccoli, garlic, lentils, mushrooms, nuts, oats, oranges, pecans, radishes, raisins, salmon, seafood, soybeans, and green leafy vegetables. Osteoporosis is one of the first signs of copper deficiency. Other signs are anemia, baldness, diarrhea, impaired breathing, and skin sores.

Essential Fatty Acids Essential fatty acids (EFAs) are necessary to improve hair texture and prevent dry, brittle hair. Fish is the best food source of EFAs.

Iron Cook in iron pots and eat more green leafy vegetables, eggs, whole-grain breads and cereals, almonds, avocados, dates, blackstrap molasses, beets, kidney and lima beans, lentils, millet, peaches, pears, prunes, pumpkin, raisins, sesame seeds, and soybeans.

Silicon Silicon is important for strong, shiny hair. Eat more alfalfa sprouts, beets, brown rice, bell peppers, soy products, green leafy vegetables, and whole grains, especially oats.

Vitamins B Find B vitamins in brown rice, egg yolks, wheat germ, whole-grain breads and cereals, peas, peanuts, poultry (aim for the organically grown to be safe), asparagus, oatmeal, plums, dried prunes, raisins, watercress, broccoli, kelp, most nuts, raw spinach, avocados, dandelion greens, leafy greens, molasses, mushrooms, carrots, tomatoes, potatoes, fish, brewer's nutritional yeast (avoid if susceptible to yeast infections), bananas, tempeh, soy beans, herring, mackerel, clams, dates, split peas, and oranges.

Vitamin C Vitamin C can improve scalp circulation. But it is not produced in the body, so you must have it daily. Sources include citrus fruits, strawberries, asparagus, avocados, beet greens, black currants, broccoli, cantaloupe, dandelion greens, kelp, mangoes, mustard greens, green peas, sweet peppers, persimmons, pineapple, radishes, spinach, Swiss chard, turnip greens, tomatoes, and watercress. High levels of vitamin C and zinc reduce copper levels. If copper intake is too high, levels of vitamin C and zinc drop. That's why it's best to get your nutrients via food.

Vitamin E Vitamin E can increase oxygen uptake and improve circulation to the scalp. Food sources include cold-pressed vegetable oils, dark green leafy vegetables, peanuts, dried beans and peas, nuts, seeds, whole grains, oatmeal, soybeans, sweet potatoes, watercress, and wheat germ.

Zinc Zinc stimulates hair growth by enhancing immune function. Food sources include egg yolks, fish, kelp, peanuts, lima beans, mushrooms, pecans, oysters, pumpkin seeds, sardines, seafood, soy beans, and sunflower seeds.

■ Headaches

There are many causes of headaches, including food allergies, stress, over- or undereating, caffeine withdrawal, exertion, and variations in estrogen levels. To find out the cause of yours, keep a food/stress diary for at least a week, but a month is better, especially if you try new foods.

Just as there are many causes, there are many types of headaches, and some of them work in concert. For example, a muscle-tension headache can increase the frequency, intensity, and duration of migraines, and vice versa.

Avoid:

Unhealthy Foods The most common foods to avoid are lunch meats that contain nitrites, fermented foods (e.g., bread, cheese, beer, and wine), MSG, artificial sweeteners, roasted nuts, chocolate, citrus juice, hard-cured sausage, pickled cabbage, alcoholic beverages, coffee, and tea. You may have your own sensitivities. Start a food/headache diary, charting what you eat and your reaction to it. Eliminate the foods that precede your headaches.

Focus On:

Fish Oil   Fish oil has a platelet-stabilizing and antispasm action that has been shown to decrease migraines. If you don't like or can't eat fish, you can get fish oil capsules at your health food store.

Low-Fat Diet   High levels of blood lipids (fats) and free fatty acids are important triggers for migraines. These triggers cause platelets to aggregate, leading to dilation of your blood vessels, a know precursor to migraines. One study undertaken to evaluate the impact of dietary fat intake on migraines and their severity was conducted over a 12-week period on 54 participants previously diagnosed with migraine headache. Each person recorded everything eaten and maintained a headache diary. The researchers found that when participants limited their dietary fat to 28 grams a day, headaches decreased in number, intensity, and duration, and less pain medication was required.

Magnesium   Magnesium is known to relax smooth muscle. Because of depleted soils, we don't get enough of this mineral in our diets. Low ionized magnesium has been linked to migraine headaches in at least one study. Unless you're eating organic vegetables, consider taking 300 mg magnesium daily (which is also good for your heart) as a preventive strategy. Older adults need 600–800 mg daily to help absorb calcium.

Tryptophan-Rich Foods   Tryptophan helps prevent headaches, so eat more foods that contain this essential amino acid. Food rich in tryptophan include brown rice, cottage cheese, turkey, peanuts, and soy protein.

Vitamin B   In one study, people who took 400 mg of riboflavin (a B vitamin) decreased the severity of their migraines by 70%. You can take B vitamins as supplements, or eat organically produced liver, chicken, peanuts, hickory nuts, soybeans, soy flour, wheat germ, whole-wheat cereal/bread/pasta, spinach, kale, peas, lima beans, sunflower seeds, and eggs. You can also find stress vitamin capsules in your health food store, pharmacy, and grocery store, which are a combination of vitamin C and B-complex vitamins.

■ Heart Disease

An article in the *Journal of the American Medicine Association* provided evidence that eating a diet low in saturated (animal) fats and high in soy, whole-wheat cereals, low-fat dairy foods, soy protein, and almonds was as effective as the drugs called *statins* in lowering cholesterol.

Avoid:

Foods and Drinks That Contribute to Heart Disease Avoid whole milk or any dairy product that is high in fat. Their consumption contributes to clogged arteries. Avoid red meat, highly spiced foods, salt, sugar, or white flour products. Refined sugars in sodas, cakes, pies, candy, cookies, doughnuts, and so forth cause wide variations in blood sugar that lead to dangerous instability in vital intracellular sugar levels. Remove coffee, black tea, colas, and other stimulants from your diet. Refrain from alcohol use.

Focus On:

Apples and Wine In a study of 34,942 postmenopausal women initially free of heart disease, apples and wine were inversely associated with coronary heart disease death. The data suggest the preventive effects of the catechins, a major group of cancer-protective flavonoids, in apples and wine. Since alcohol is a hot flash trigger, try eating more grapes, including the seeds and skins.

Calcium Calcium can reduce palpitations and high blood pressure. It also protects the heart. Calcium comes in many forms, some more absorbable than others. Probably the most absorbable form comes from eating a diet rich in calcium that includes daily amounts of one or more of the following foods:

almonds	dulse (seaweed)	peppermint
asparagus	fennel	prunes
blackstrap molasses	figs	salmon with bones
broccoli	filberts	sardines
buttermilk	flaxseeds	seafood
cabbage	goat's milk	sesame seeds
carob	kale	tofu
cheese (soy)	kelp	turnip greens
chickory	mustard greens	watercress
collards	oats	
dandelion greens	parsley	

Carotenes   Carotenes are associated with a lower risk of heart disease, especially coronary artery disease in women. One study followed 73,286 female nurses and their consumption of foods. The ones who ate the highest levels of dietary carotenoids had the lowest risk of coronary artery disease. Foods to eat to reduce your chance of coronary artery disease include carrots, broccoli, turnip greens, beets, spinach, parsley, yellow squash, garlic, papaya, and cantaloupe.

Flaxseed   Flaxseed is good for your heart because it has the right kind of heart-healthy oil in it. (See Hot Flashes for more information on how to use flaxseed.)

Lycopene   Lycopene is a nutrient found in tomatoes, tomato products (even ketchup!), and fruits such as watermelon. The Women's Health Study showed that lycopene can prevent heart disease in women. More than 40,000 women were tracked for 11 years. Those who ate the most tomato-based products reduced their risk of heart disease by 33%. The daily therapeutic amount appears to be about 20 mg, which is twice the amount in the average American diet. Lycopene is also available in a supplement form.

Magnesium   Magnesium deficiency is believed to have adverse heart and blood vessel consequences, including high blood pressure (hypertension), diabetes, palpitations (arrhythmias), heart attack, and hardening of the arteries (atherosclerosis). A recent study provided evidence that participants who consumed the lowest amounts of magnesium were twice as likely to develop heart disease as those who consumed the highest amount. Magnesium-rich foods include whole-grain bread and cereals, peas, soy, wheat germ, nuts, figs, and green leafy vegetables, such as spinach and kale.

Maitake Mushrooms   The versatile maitake mushroom is an *adaptogen*—a substance that helps the body maintain equilibrium. It helps maintain healthy blood pressure and cholesterol levels, and can be found or ordered from your local supermarket or health food store.

Nuts   According to a study in the *Archives of Internal Medicine*, adults who ate 1 ounce of nuts (such as walnuts or almonds) at least twice a week had a 47% lower risk of sudden cardiac death and a 30% lower risk of heart disease compared to those who ate no nuts. Another study in *Circulation* showed almonds used as snacks in the meal plans of people with high cholesterol significantly reduced coronary heart disease risk factors.

Potassium   Potassium deficiency represents a risk for heart palpitations. Eat foods high in potassium including spinach, cabbage, cauliflower, tomatoes, carrots, soy, and wheat germ.

Soy   The Food and Drug Administration's ruling on soy labels allows products that have at least 6.25 grams of soy protein per serving to carry this label: "Twenty-five grams of soy protein a day, as part of a diet low in saturated fat and cholesterol, may reduce the risk of heart disease."

Which foods have the most soy protein? Probably the supplemental form, but it may provide a too concentrated form of isoflavones, so concentrate on the following foods:

½ cup soy nuts = 39 g

½ cup tempeh = 19 g

4 oz. firm tofu = 13

8 oz. plain soy milk = 10

1 soy-based burger = 10–12 g

4 oz. soft or silken tofu = 9 g

(*Source*: The United Soybean Board)

Your best bet is probably tempeh because it doesn't contain the phytates that other soy does, which interfere with the absorption of some minerals, including zinc. Choose the organic form.

Tryptophan-Rich Foods Tryptophan is good for the heart, so eat more foods that contain this essential amino acid. Foods rich in tryptophan include brown rice, cottage cheese, turkey, peanuts, and soy protein.

Vitamin B6 and Folate A large study by Brigham and Women's Hospital at the Harvard School of Public Health suggests that women with the highest intake of vitamin B6 (pyridoxine) and folate (folic acid) cut their heart disease risk in half compared to women with the lowest intake. Food sources of vitamin B6 include brewer's nutritional yeast, carrots, eggs, fish, meat, peas, spinach, sunflower seeds, walnuts, wheat germ, avocados, bananas, beans, blackstrap molasses, broccoli, brown rice and other whole grains, cabbage, cantaloupe, corn, dulse, plantains, potatoes, rice bran, soybeans, and tempeh. Foods that contain folic acid include barley, bran, brewer's nutritional yeast, brown rice, dates, green leafy vegetables, legumes (peanuts, dried peas, and beans), lentils, mushrooms, oranges, split peas, root vegetables, salmon, tuna, and wheat germ, and whole-grain cereal and breads. Avoid nutritional yeast if susceptible to yeast infections.

Vitamin B12 Palpitations can be caused by a deficiency of vitamin B12. Food sources for this vitamin are brewer's nutritional yeast, clams, eggs, herring, kidney, liver, mackerel, seafood, sea vegetables (dulse, kelp, kombu, and nori), soybeans, and soy products.

Vitamin C Using the information from the Nurse's Study of 85,118 female nurses, a group of researchers examined the relationship between vitamin C and risk for coronary heart disease (CHD). They found the users of vitamin C supplements had the lowest risk for CHD, followed by the women who received their vitamin C from diet alone. Sources of vitamin C include alfalfa sprouts asparagus, avocados, beet greens, black currants, broccoli, brussels sprouts, cabbage, cantaloupe, collards, dandelion greens, dulse (sea vegetable), grapefruit, kale, lemons, mangoes, mustard greens, onions, oranges, papayas, green peas, sweet peppers, persimmons, pineapple, radish, rose hips, spinach, strawberries, Swiss chard, tomatoes, turnip greens, and watercress.

Vitamins D and K In a randomized placebo-controlled study, 181 postmenopausal women were given either a placebo (sugar pill) or a supplement containing minerals and vitamin D or the same supplement with vitamin K. The group receiving a supplement containing either vitamin D or vitamin K had a beneficial effect on the elastic properties of their artery walls. Eating foods high in vitamin D (eggs, salmon, tuna) and/or K (spinach, cabbage, cauliflower, tomatoes, carrots, soy, wheat germ) may also be helpful. Cod liver oil is also an important source of vitamin D.

Whole Grains Eating more whole-grain foods has been related to a reduced risk of developing diabetes and heart disease. Eating whole-grain breads, cereals, and pastas can reduce your risk of heart disease.

■ Hot Flashes

Avoid:

Triggering Foods Hot flashes are often triggered by external factors such as alcohol, caffeine, sugary food, hot foods and/or hot beverages. As a start, remove these items from your menu.

Focus On:

Flaxseed   Flaxseed may be a good bet for you if you have mild menopausal symptoms. A study completed at Laval University in Quebec and published in *Obstetrics and Gynecology* found that taking flaxseed can successfully treat mild menopausal symptoms as successfully as taking hormones. This held for women whether they'd had a hysterectomy or experienced natural menopause. The reduction in symptoms didn't seem to be related to diet, exercise, or weight. If you're diabetic, flaxseed can also lower your glucose and insulin levels.

Flaxseed can be found at health food stores and is inexpensive. Put a handful of seeds in your blender and they will reduce to a powder in a minute or two. (If you don't have a blender, you can buy flaxseed in powder form, but it's more expensive.) Add a tablespoon or so to your morning breakfast cereal, glass of tomato juice, soup, smoothie, or cup of yogurt, or sprinkle it on your salad. It has a nutty, clean taste. I have a client who puts flaxseed powder in a glass of water, stirs, and drinks it down. Because it is a fiber and absorbs liquid, take it with plenty of noncaffeinated liquids. Have flaxseed daily for at least 2 months to achieve maximum benefits.

Soy   A double-blind, randomized, placebo-controlled trial of 104 women aged 45 to 62 found that those who ate 60 grams of soy protein (two to three servings) daily for 12 weeks experienced a 45% reduction in hot flashes. Another study used a questionnaire to query 1,106 menopausal women about their soy intake. Whether women took hormones or not, the more soy foods they ate, the more they reduced the severity of their hot flashes; smoking increased the risk of flashes. The women who had the greatest relief from hot flashes averaged three servings a day: the equivalent of 12 ounces of tofu or three 8-ounce glasses of soy milk.

In a review of all the studies completed (19) involving more than 1,700 women, there was a statistically significant relationship between initial hot flash frequency and soy foods or isoflavone supplements. This means soy reduces hot flashes.

Soy has played a prominent role in other cultures for centuries. According to the *Harvard Women's Health Watch*, observational evidence indicates the benefits of a diet rich in soy far outweigh the risks. The traditional Asian diet contains 30 to 50 mg daily of isoflavones. Research studies have usually tested daily doses varying from 40 to 80 mg. If you plan to try soy, aim for approximately a cup of soy milk, one-half cup of roasted soy nuts, or 4 ounces of tempeh daily.

Vitamin E   Vitamin E is an especially good choice to reduce hot flashes if you can't take estrogen. Estrogen can stimulate the growth of breast cancer cells, but vitamin E doesn't. In a study at the Mayo Clinic, Dr. Charles L. Loprinzi asked 120 breast cancer survivors to take 800 I.U. of vitamin E daily for 4 weeks, followed by a placebo for another 4 weeks. While the women were taking the vitamin E, they had a decrease in hot flashes.

■ Insomnia/Sleep Problems

Avoid:

Alcohol   Avoid drinking alcohol at night. It can impede sleep.

Caffeine   Caffeinated beverages are associated with insomnia, so if you must drink them, do so before 4 P.M.

Sugary Foods   Sugar raises your blood glucose level abruptly, then lowers it, interfering with sleep. Eating chocolate or drinking colas can be especially bad because they contain both sugar and caffeine.

Focus on:

Biotin   A biotin deficiency can lead to insomnia. To ward off sleep problems, eat more brewer's nutritional yeast, cooked egg yolks, poultry, saltwater fish, soybeans, and whole grains.

Calcium   Calcium may aid sleep and rest. Calcium comes in many forms, some more adsorbable than others. Probably the most adsorbable form comes from eating a diet rich in calcium that includes daily amounts of one or more of the following foods:

almonds	dulse (seaweed)	parsley
asparagus	fennel	peppermint
blackstrap molasses	figs	prunes
broccoli	filberts	salmon with bones
buttermilk	flaxseeds	sardines
cabbage	goat's milk	seafood
carob	green leafy vegetables	sesame seeds
cheese (soy)	kale	tofu
chickory	kelp	turnip greens
collards	mustard greens	watercress
dandelion greens	oats	

Folic Acid   Insomnia and sleep problems (including restless leg syndrome—those creepy, crawling, pulling leg sensations) can be a sign of folic acid deficiency. To protect against fatigue, eat more barley, brewer's nutritional yeast, brown rice, chicken, dates, green leafy vegetables, legumes, lentils, liver, mushrooms, oranges, split peas, root vegetables, salmon, tuna, wheat germ, and whole-grain cereals and breads.

Magnesium   Magnesium is needed to regulate sleep. This mineral works with calcium to help you sleep. Magnesium-rich foods include whole-grain bread and cereals, peas, soy, wheat germ, nuts, figs, and green leafy vegetables such as spinach and kale.

Melatonin-Rich Foods   Banana, cucumber, beets, and rice contain melatonin, an antioxidant that protects tissues and aids in sleep. Fill up on one or more of these foods at dinner.

Tryptophan-Rich Foods   Tryptophan is a building block of protein necessary for the production of vitamin B3 (niacin). It is used by the brain to produce serotonin, a neurotransmitter that transfers nerve impulses from cell to cell and is responsible for sleep. Foods rich in tryptophan include brown rice, cottage cheese, turkey, peanuts, and soy protein.

■ Itchiness

Avoid:

Foods That Make You Itch   Rule out food allergies and sensitivities. Keep a food/itchiness journal and you'll begin to see patterns. Once you make a connection between a food and itchiness, stop eating it for a couple of weeks to clear it from your system. If you have a minor to moderate sensitivity, you may be able to eat the food once every 4 days, but only time and your food/itchiness journal will tell.

Focus On:

Fatty Acids   Taking fish oil can reduce itchiness, according to a study at Purdue University reported in the *American Journal of Clinical Nutrition*. If you're itching, have sardines or Spanish mackerel at your next meal and see if it helps.

Flaxseeds or Sunflower Seeds   Although the research carried out at Texas A&M University used skin and hair coats in dogs, the results may be helpful to humans, too. A month-long supplementation with either flaxseed or sunflower seed provided improvement in skin.

Drinking More Water   Itching and dry skin can be due to dehydration, especially if you're having hot flashes, feeling stress, and sweating a lot. Be sure to drink 8–10 glasses daily of either distilled water or water that has been run through a reverse osmosis filter. You can buy this kind of filter at a health food store or online.

■ Joint and Muscle Pain

Avoid:

Vitamins and Mineral Depletion Insufficient intake of fruits, vegetables and whole grains, sweating, stress, lack of activity, smoking, alcohol, illness and more can deplete your body of the vitamins and minerals needed for strong, healthy joints and mussles.

Focus On:

Calcium Calcium can relieve muscle spasms and pain. Calcium comes in many forms, some more absorbable than others. Probably the most absorbable form comes from eating a diet that includes daily amounts of one or more of the following foods:

almonds	dulse (seaweed)	peppermint
asparagus	fennel	prunes
blackstrap molasses	figs	salmon with bones
broccoli	filberts	sardines
buttermilk	flaxseeds	seafood
cabbage	goat's milk	sesame seeds
carob	kale	tofu
cheese (soy)	kelp	turnip greens
chickory	mustard greens	watercress
collards	oats	whey
dandelion greens	parsley	yogurt

Magnesium Magnesium works with calcium to relax muscles and make healthy bones. Magnesium-rich foods include whole-grain bread and cereals, peas, soy, wheat germ, nuts, figs, green leafy vegetables, spinach, and kale.

■ Memory Loss and Foggy Thinking

Avoid:

Alcohol   Alcohol can deplete many B vitamins that are essential for healthy memory and brain function.

Caffeine   Too much caffeine from coffee, colas, and even chocolate can negatively affect your memory function.

Dieting   Most women are regular dieters and either starve themselves or follow diets that deprive the brain of an adequate supply of proteins, fats, and carbohydrates necessary for optimal brain function.

Sugar   Any food with sugar in it can lead to poor concentration and memory lapses. A study at New York University published in the *Proceedings of the National Academy of Sciences* found that middle-aged and elderly adults with impairment in glucose tolerance had a small hippocampus—the brain region so crucial for recent memory. The good news is that if you get off the sugary foods and start to exercise, you can protect your brain. Even artificial sweeteners such as aspartame can cause toxic reactions in your body that show up as memory loss.

Focus On:

Blueberries   Blueberries have been shown both by experiment and through collecting information about foods and their effect on memory to be protective of the cognitive (thinking) functions.

Green Tea   Both experimental and epidemiological evidence demonstrates that flavonoid polyphenols, particularly from green tea, improve age-related cognitive (memory and thinking) processes.

Olive Oil   The *monounsaturated fats* of the olive oil–rich Mediterranean diet can help maintain clear thinking, according to researchers at the University of Bari in Italy. They reported their findings in the May 1999 issue of the journal *Neurology*. They observed 278 older adults who had consumed diets high in monoun-saturated fatty acids chiefly from extra-virgin olive oil. They found the oil protected the older adults from age-related cognitive decline. The researchers theorized the olive oil helps bolster the structure of brain cell membranes. Participants received more than 17% of their daily calories from monounsaturated fats, 85% of which came from olive oil. If you're cooking or making a salad dressing, choose extra-virgin olive oil.

Sprouts, Kidney Beans, Eggs, and Whole Grains Research find-ings suggest that even a minor iron deficiency can be hazardous to your memory. Good sources of iron include alfalfa sprouts, kidney beans, eggs, and whole-grain cereals and breads. Be sure you get enough iron-rich foods.

Calcium Calcium can improve memory. The mineral comes in many forms, some more absorbable than others. Probably the most absorbable form comes from eating a diet that includes daily amounts of one or more of the following foods:

almonds	dulse (seaweed)	parsley
asparagus	fennel	peppermint
blackstrap molasses	figs	prunes
broccoli	filberts	salmon with bones
buttermilk	flaxseeds	sardines
cabbage	goat's milk	seafood
carob	green leafy vegetables	sesame seeds
cheese (soy)	kale	tofu
chickory	kelp	turnip greens
collards	mustard greens	watercress
dandelion greens	oats	

Choline Choline is a building block for the neurotransmitter acetylcholine. Without adequate levels of this substance, the brain can't store or retrieve information. Brewer's nutritional yeast (avoid if prone to yeast infections) and wheat germ are some of the richest sources of choline.

Folic Acid   Memory loss can be a sign of folic acid deficiency. Eat more barley, brewer's nutritional yeast (avoid if prone to yeast infections), brown rice, chicken, dates, green leafy vegetables, legumes, lentils, liver, mushrooms, oranges, split peas, root vegetables, salmon, tuna, wheat germ, and whole-grain cereals and breads.

Vitamin B6   Pyridoxine deficiency can lead to memory loss. Food sources include brewer's nutritional yeast (avoid if prone to yeast infections), carrots, chicken, eggs, fish, peas, spinach, sunflower seeds, walnuts, wheat germ, avocados, bananas, beans, blackstrap molasses, broccoli, brown rice and other whole grains, cabbage, cantaloupe, corn, dulse, plantains, potatoes, soybeans, and tempeh.

Vitamin C and Beta-Carotene Foods   A study of 6,400 older adults found that ascorbic acid and beta-carotene were significant predictors of improved free recall, vocabulary, and recognition—all memory functions. Food sources of vitamin C include citrus fruits, green peppers, strawberries, broccoli, cauliflower, parsley, watercress, cabbage, onions, alfalfa sprouts, and raw spinach. Sources of beta-carotene include carrots, broccoli, turnip greens, oranges, grapefruit, beets, raw spinach, parsley, yellow squash, garlic, papaya, and cantaloupe.

Supplements   If after cutting out sugar, alcohol, caffeine, and processed foods, and adding memory-enhancing foods, your memory is still foggy, you may want to consider supplements. Elisa Lottor, ND, recommends the following daily brain-boosting supplements along with a multivitamin/mineral formula. Start slowly at the lowest dose and add them one at a time in the order listed. Use vitamin B-complex for several weeks, keeping track of your memory in a memory/supplement diary. If your memory is still fuzzy, add the next supplement.

• The B-complex vitamins are key nutrients for a healthy nervous system. Stress depletes the body of B-complex vitamins.

Choose a combination with 25 milligrams or more for individual B vitamins, 400 micrograms and up for folic acid, and 25 micrograms and up for vitamin B12.

• Vitamin E in mixed tocopherol form protects the fatty tissue of the brain and slows down the progression of Alzheimer's disease. Take 400 I.U. and up. The results of a study of 3,385 Japanese-Americans in Hawaii showed that vitamin E and C supplements taken alone or together resulted in improved thinking ability.

• Essential fatty acids from fish-liver oil. Fish-liver oil is rich in omega-3 fatty acids, which are important antiinflammatories that enhance chemical brain processes associated with memory and learning.

■ Menstrual Bleeding

Nutrition is an important factor in erratic perimenopausal bleeding. Eating red meat and dairy products may cause or contribute to hormonal imbalance and bleeding. Unstable blood sugar levels are an important factor, too. Food allergies can also contribute as well as vitamin and/or mineral deficiencies and depressed mood.

Avoid:

Red Meat, Dairy Products, Sodas, and Caffeine Dairy products block the absorption of magnesium. Eating red meat and dairy products promotes hormonal imbalance due to excessive estrogen and inadequate progesterone levels. Meat also contains an abundance of *methianine,* an amino acid that promotes inflammation and elevated *homocysteine.* An elevation in homocysteine indicates the body's immunologic system has failed. At the very least, limit animal protein to three or four servings a week—lean meat and fish are best. Cut out sugary treats because they also make it hard for your body to absorb magnesium. Caffeine and alcohol push calcium and other important nutrients out of your body because they act as diuretics. In one study, women who consumed caffeine (coffee, chocolate, caffeinated sodas or tea) were four times more likely than others to have severe PMS. Keep a food/mood/bleeding journal and see what affects you.

Focus On:

Calcium   If you're not eating dairy foods, eat more broccoli, soy products, fish (especially sardines and salmon with the bones), tomatoes, whole-wheat bread, molasses, almonds, and green leafy vegetables. If you decide to take a calcium/magnesium supplement, make sure it's of the citrate variety so that it will be better absorbed. (See Breast Cancer, Calcium-Rich Foods, and Memory Loss, this chapter, for more information.)

Calcium is important for strong bones. It also calms nerves and is necessary for keeping your muscles working, making the glue *(collagen)* that holds your body together and transporting nutrients in and out of your cells. You need vitamin D to absorb calcium, so be sure you expose your face and arms to least 15 minutes of sunlight a day. That will uplift your mood as well. If you live in the north, you probably aren't getting enough sunlight unless you go for a walk on your lunch hour or take cod liver oil (high in vitamins A and D) daily.

Complex Carbohydrates   Complex carbohydrates can reduce stress and assist in healing after perimenopausal bleeding. Complex carbohydrates are whole fruits and vegetables, whole-grain bread, cereals, pasta, dried beans, and peas. They take a long time to digest and keep your blood sugar up. Researchers speculate that such a diet may increase your body's *serotonin,* a brain chemical with anti-depressant properties.

Fruits and Vegetables   Get at least five servings of fresh or frozen, preferably organically grown, fruits and vegetables a day. These foods will not only enhance your health but will help replace blood lost through perimenopausal bleeding because they are full of fluid, minerals, and vitamins.

Iron   Replace the iron you're losing through bleeding. Instead of a supplement, many of which aren't well absorbed, try eating more iron-rich foods like prunes, raisins, purple grapes, kidney beans, alfalfa sprouts, molasses (one tablespoon of blackstrap molasses twice a day), egg yolks, and whole-grain breads and cereals. Use powdered kelp and garlic in cooking to provide needed minerals and to help you heal after excessive bleeding. The two best ways to replenish lost iron are to cook with iron pots and eat iron-rich foods.

Vitamins E and B Complex Eat foods high in vitamins E and B complex to provide energy, balance hormones, relieve stress, and promote blood cell productivity. Eat several of these foods daily: sunflower seeds, wheat germ, whole-wheat breads and cereals, rolled oats, asparagus, brown rice, raisins, lima beans, soy burgers, tempeh, salmon, prunes, lentils, peanuts, tuna, white beans, bananas, walnuts, sweet potatoes, sardines, crab, herring, trout, mackerel.

Vitamin K Vitamin K helps with normal blood clotting. Foods to focus on include wheat germ, alfalfa sprouts, raw spinach, cabbage, cauliflower, tomatoes, baked or steamed potatoes, carrots, and peas.

■ Osteoporosis

Avoid:

Animal Protein, Sugar, and Salt Animal protein, sugar, and salt cause your body to excrete increased amounts of calcium. Reduce your intake of these three items.

Caffeine and Alcohol Caffeine and alcohol leach minerals, including calcium, from your body.

Sodas and Processed Foods Too much phosphorus, which is found in most sodas and many processed foods, steals calcium from your bones. Choose water, herbal tea, or diluted fresh fruit juice.

Calcium Calcium intake can have an impact on whether you have osteoporosis and how severe it is. If you are premenopausal, get 1,000 mg a day. If you are postmenopausal, take 1,500 mg a day. You can obtain calcium from food sources, usually about 500 mg, from foods such as broccoli, whole-grain breads and cereals, fish (eat the bones of sardines and salmon and the shells of shrimp), sprouts, and dark green leafy vegetables like raw spinach and kale.

Iron   Iron is an important nutrient associated with bone health. Collagen, an integral component of bone, cannot be produced without it. A recent study of menopausal women found that those who consumed 18 mg iron a day, along with adequate calcium (1,500 mg a day), had the greatest bone mineral density.

Caffeine, a high intake of high-fiber foods, and calcium supplements can reduce iron absorption. If you take iron in a supplement, take it separately from calcium or calcium-rich foods. Vitamin C slightly increases iron absorption. Taking vitamin A with iron helps treat iron deficiency, since vitamin A helps the body use iron stored in the liver.

Since heme iron from meat is associated with heart disease and iron supplements are not well absorbed, your best bet might be to obtain sufficient iron daily from nonheme iron sources. Combine some of the following foods to obtain your daily quotient of 18 mg iron:

1 cup soy flour = 8.8 mg

1 cup wheat germ = 5.5 mg

⅓ cup sesame seeds = 5.2 mg

¼ cup brewer's nutritional yeast = 5 mg (avoid if prone to yeast infections)

2 tablespoons blackstrap (unrefined) molasses = 4.6 mg

1 cup brown rice = 4 mg

⅓ cup sunflower seeds = 3.5 mg

½ cup almonds = 3.3 mg

½ cup unsalted cashews, = 2.9 mg

1 cup bean soup = 2.8 mg

1 cup macaroni and cheese = 2.6 mg

1 cup spaghetti with tomatoes and cheese = 2 mg

½ cup baked beans = 2 mg

1 cup yellow cornmeal = 1.8 mg

10 dried apricots = 1.7 mg

1 cup oatmeal = 1.7 mg

10 dates = 1.6 mg

½ cup raw English walnuts = 1.5 mg

1 cup split pea soup = 1.4 mg

2 slices whole-wheat bread = 1.4 mg

4 buckwheat or whole-wheat pancakes (4 in.) = 1.3 mg

3 oz. turkey = 1.2 mg

1 raw stalk broccoli = 1.1 mg

3 oz. tuna in water = 1.0 mg

¼ cup raisins = 1.0 mg

If you don't eat enough of these foods, cook in iron pots and pans to obtain your iron.

Magnesium Magnesium can aid in protecting you against osteoporosis. Magnesium-rich foods include whole-grain bread and cereals, peas, soy, wheat germ, nuts, figs, green leafy vegetables, spinach, and kale.

Onions Onions have been found to increase bone mass in several studies. Eating more onions will strengthen your bones and guard against osteoporosis. Steamed, raw, baked, broiled—you have many options.

Soy At the end of a study of postmenopausal women who for 6 months consumed 40 grams a day of isolated soy protein that contained 2.24 mg isoflavones per grain, significant increases were noted in bone mineral content and density in the lumbar spine as well as an increase in HDL ("good") cholesterol. Another study using 54 mg/day of the dietary phytoestrogen genistein (one of the isoflavones in soy) turned out to be as effective as hormone therapy in stopping menopause-related bone loss without causing side effects. A third study provided evidence that soy contributes to the low risk of osteoporosis in Asian women. To provide additional support for your bones, eat more soy. Choose from tofu, tempeh, soy cheese, soy milk, and soy hot dogs. You may even find soy lunch meats at your grocery store. Choose the organic form.

Focus On:

Vitamin B-Complex   B vitamins are known to reduce levels of homocysteine, an amino acid that doubles the risk of osteoporosis-related fractures, according to Dr. Douglas P. Kiel, senior author of a study that appeared in the *New England Journal of Medicine*. Homocysteine may interfere with crucial chemical bonds within the bones. Kiel said that a standard multivitamin taken once a day will bring your homocysteine levels below the danger point. Foods naturally rich in B vitamins can also reduce your risk of broken bones, including broccoli and other green leafy vegetables, carrots, avocados, cantaloupes, apricots, almonds and peanuts, sunflower seeds, oats, green peas, soy, lima beans, wheat germ, grapes, eggs, salmon, tuna, cooked cabbage, walnuts, mackerel, mushrooms, and cauliflower.

■ Reduced Sex Drive or Intercourse Discomfort

After menopause the vagina can thin and shorten, making intercourse uncomfortable.

Avoid:

A Diet Focused on Fruits, Sugar, and Yeast   Avoid aged cheeses, alcohol, chocolate, dried fruits, fermented foods, wheat, oats, rye and barley, ham, honey, nut butters, pickles, raw mushrooms, soy sauce, sugar in any form, vinegar, and all products containing yeast. Also eliminate citrus and acidic fruits (oranges, grapefruits, lemons, tomatoes, pineapple, and limes) until inflammation or discomfort abates. Add them back one at a time, noting how the food affects your intercourse discomfort.

Focus On:

Foods with Estrogen-Like Activity   Foods with estrogen-like activity can help strengthen vaginal walls. Eat more alfalfa sprouts, other beans (mung, red, split peas, etc.), apples, and oily seeds

Oats   The unripe oat grain is used as an antidepressant and as a restorative nerve tonic to relieve stress and exhaustion. Australian researchers found that athletes who followed an oat-based diet for 3 weeks showed a 4% increase in stamina. Start eating whole-grain oat cereal at least once a day and see what happens.

Soy   In a 2003 study, researchers analyzed the effects of a 6-month soy-rich diet on the vaginal lining of 187 postmenopausal women in a randomized clinical trial. The researchers found the soy diet was as effective as hormone therapy in preventing vaginal atrophy, which could go a long way toward reducing intercourse discomfort.

■ Skin Problems

Avoid:

Detrimental Food and Drinks   Avoid fried foods, animal fats, and heat-processed vegetable oils. Beware of any oils that have been subjected to high heat during processing or cooking. Heating oils produces free radicals, which have a destructive effect on the skin. Avoid drinking soft drinks or eating sugar, chocolate, potato chips, or other junk foods that provide nutritive value. Avoid alcohol and caffeine. The diuretic effect of these substances causes cells, including those in the skin, to lose fluids and essential minerals.

Focus On:

Biotin   Sufficient quantities of biotin are needed for healthy skin. Food sources to include in your meal plans are brewer's nutritional yeast (unless prone to yeast infections), cooked egg yolks, poultry, saltwater fish, soybeans, and whole-grain breads and cereals.

Calcium A deficiency in calcium contributes to fragility of the skin. Calcium comes in many forms, some more absorbable than others. Probably the most absorbable form comes from eating a diet that includes daily amounts of one or more of the following foods:

almonds	dulse (seaweed)	peppermint
asparagus	fennel	prunes
blackstrap molasses	figs	salmon with bones
broccoli	filberts	sardines
buttermilk	flaxseeds	seafood
cabbage	goat's milk	sesame seeds
carob	kale	tofu
cheese (soy)	kelp	turnip greens
chickory	mustard greens	watercress
collards	oats	whey
dandelion greens	parsley	yogurt

Fish Oil, Flaxseeds, and Sunflower Seeds Studies reported in the *American Journal of Clinical Nutrition* and *Veterinary Dermatology* provide evidence that n-3 fatty acids, found in fish (sardines, Spanish mackerel, tuna), fish oil capsules, flaxseeds, and sunflower seeds can improve skin health and itching.

Multivitamins and Minerals Dr. Sarah Brewer, iVillages' resident expert for gynecological and women's health, suggests taking a multivitamin and mineral supplement that provides 100% of the Recommended Dietary Allowance (RDA) of as many micronutrients as possible plus important trace elements such as chromium, copper, boron, and molybdenum.

Vitamin B6 Vitamin B6 (pyridoxine) deficiency can lead to flaky skin. Food sources include brewer's nutritional yeast, carrots, chicken, eggs, fish, peas, spinach, sunflower seeds, walnuts, wheat germ, avocados, bananas, beans, blackstrap molasses, broccoli, brown rice and other whole grains, cabbage, cantaloupe, corn, dulse, plantains, potatoes, soybeans, and tempeh.

■ Urinary Symptoms

After menopause, your urinary apparatus thins and is more susceptible to infection and irritation.

Avoid:

Foods and Drugs That Irritate the Bladder   Diets linked to alcohol,
tomatoes, spices, chocolate, caffeinated and citrus beverages, and
high-acid foods can worsen bladder irritation. Some women find all
fruits, especially fruit juices, irritating. If that's the case, consider taking cranberry extract in tablet or liquid form, following the label in-
structions for dosage. Chemicals in drugs and impure water can have
an adverse effect on the bladder. Avoid taking excess zinc and iron
supplements until you're healed. Taking more than 100 mg zinc daily
can depress your immune system. Bacteria require iron to grow.
When you have an infection, your body stores iron in your spleen,
liver, and bone marrow to reduce the growth of bacteria. Food allergies can mimic bladder infections. Keep a food/bladder infection diary
to see if you can find connections between problems and your diet.

Focus On:

Basil   Basil is a sweet herb you can use in salads, soups,
casseroles, and other main dishes. It has been shown to control the
growth and survival of *Escherichia coli* (the major cause of bladder
infections), *Staphylococcus aureus, Yersinia enterocolitica, Pseudomonas aeruginosa, Lactobacillus plantarum, Aspergillus niger,* Geotrichum, and Rhodotorula.

Blueberries   Recent research at Rutgers University in New Jersey
found that blueberries can effectively prevent urinary tract infections
(UTIs). Blueberries contain compounds called *proanthocyanidins*
that keep *E. coli* (the bacteria responsible for most UTIs) from at-
taching to the cells in the walls of the urinary tract. A generous hand-

ful of blueberries a day will help prevent bladder infections and maintain urinary tract health.

Coriander Use this spice in sweet dishes. Coriander has been shown to control the growth and survival of *Escherichia coli, Staphylococcus aureus, Yersinia enterocolitica, Pseudomonas aeruginosa, Lactobacillus plantarum, Aspergillus niger,* Geotrichum, and Rhodotorula.

Cranberries According to folk medicine, cranberry juice stops bladder infections. Researchers studied 150 women with UTIs and found that a glass of low-sugar cranberry juice a day is all that is needed to keep these infections away. An analysis of all well-designed studies of cranberry juice and cranberry tablets found there was no difference in the effectiveness between them. Cranberry juice can decrease the number of UTIs over a 12-month period in women, but many participants dropped out of the studies, indicating cranberry juice may not be acceptable over long periods of time.

Oregano Use this herb in salads, soups, casseroles, and other main dishes. Oregano has been shown to control the growth and survival of *E. coli* (the major cause of bladder infections), *Staphylococcus aureus, Yersinia enterocolitica, Pseudomonas aeruginosa, Lactobacillus plantarum, Aspergillus niger,* Geotrichum, and Rhodotorula.

Pineapple Fresh pineapple has enzymes called *bromelains* that have an anti-inflammatory effect on the urinary tract.

Sulfur-Rich Foods Sulfur is a mineral that may help with bladder disorders. Foods high in sulfur include cabbage, brussels sprouts, peas, cauliflower, eggs, onions, and asparagus.

Water and Vegetable Juices Dr. David Williams, editor of *Alternatives Newsletter,* says that if everyone drank 8 glasses of water every day and 1 pint of raw carrot juice with 1 pint of raw spinach juice (1 quart of juice combined), "most urologists would be out of business."

Adding celery or parsley juice to carrot juice is especially good because these juices are natural cleansers. If you don't have a juicer, you can make juice in a blender by blending the vegetables very finely while adding just 1 cup of distilled water. After blending, strain the liquid and drink immediately. If you have recurring or persistent urinary problems, a juicer may be a good purchase.

Watermelon Eat watermelon by itself at least an hour after or before eating any other food. Watermelon can help cleanse your kidneys and bladder.

■ Weight Gain

Why is it so hard to lose weight and keep it off? One study shows that weight loss causes metabolic changes that actually work to get you back to your former weight. This is why dieting isn't a good idea. Your body perceives your action as a signal to go into starvation mode and use calories more efficiently. The best way to lose weight is to follow a healthy nutritional plan focused on nutrient-rich foods and exercise every day.

Avoid:

Sugary Foods A study in the *Journal of the American Dietetic Association* concluded that in a group of men and women who ate the same number of calories, the ones who ate refined sugars (pies, cakes, and so forth as opposed to natural sugars in fruits) gained more weight. Eating sugary foods that are also high in fat puts on even more weight because the foods taste good, yet are not satisfying. This leads to eating more and more cookies, candy bars, doughnuts, cakes, pies, ice cream, Danish or sweet rolls, and other baked goods according to studies in *Nutrition Reports* and *International Journal of Eating Disorders.*

Processed Foods Processed foods (as opposed to whole foods like vegetables, fruits, seeds, and nuts) don't have enough fiber in them to keep blood glucose levels low. Consuming too many processed foods can produce insulin resistance and send blood glucose to fat depositories on your hips, thighs, buttocks, and wherever else you gain weight.

Meat and Animal Products Reduce or eliminate meat and animal products that stress your kidneys and liver and leave more room for the fruits, vegetables, and grains you need to stay healthy and lose weight. A vegetarian eating plan is associated with reduced risk of heart disease, diabetes, and other chronic illness, and lower weight, according to studies in *Public Health Nutrition, American Journal of Clinical Nutrition,* and *Preventive Medicine.*

Salt Salt makes your body get rid of helpful calcium. Use kelp (a sea vegetable that contains all the sea's mineral salts) instead, as it has been shown to increase thyroid function, which can help with weight loss.

Eating Too Fast and Eating Too Much at Night Never do anything else while you're eating so you can listen to your fullness signals and stop eating when you're full. Eating light all day but having a large meal at night causes people to store more fat according to a study in *Medicine and Science in Sports and Exercise.* Even participants who reduced their daily calories and exercised vigorously could not lose weight, and some even gained weight, when they ate a heavy meal at night or snacked after dinner.

Focus On:

Flaxseed Because it is a seed, flaxseed adds fiber to your diet. You will be more regular and your body will flush out toxins (pesticides, heavy metals, remnants of drugs or alcohol, etc.) more easily if you eat flaxseeds. If you want to lose weight, fiber fills you up, so you will feel satisfied.

Drinking Enough Water Drink 2 quarts of distilled water from the grocery store or water that has been filtered through a reverse osmosis system. You can buy a system from health food stores or online. Drink a glass of water when you get hungry and before a meal. It also fills you up so you don't overeat.

Eating Breakfast When you skip a meal, your metabolism slows and your body starts to go into starvation mode. For best results, eat four to six small meals throughout the day.

Eating Lots of Vegetables and Fruits Eat a rainbow of vegetables (three to five servings) and fruits (two to three servings) every day, preferably from local organic farms that use composting methods. These foods have the highest nutrient content and the greatest enzyme activity. They can fill you up, satisfy you, help digest your food.

If you don't like to eat veggies or think they are too expensive, research presented at the 2003 American Heart Association's scientific forum may sway you. Their findings suggest that the healthier you eat, the lower your medical costs later in life. Eating veggies can actually save you money down the road! Participants in the study with high vegetable intake (at least 42 cups a month) had the lowest annual Medicare charges, while those in the low-intake group (under 14 cups of vegetables a month) had the highest. Previous studies have linked those in the high-intake group to a lower risk of death from heart disease, stroke, and cancer.

Train your taste buds to like vegetables. If you're hungry, they'll taste good, especially if you dribble olive oil on them and shake on some garlic powder, basil, and thyme, or your favorite spices. Try them with salsa or soy mayonnaise! Hide them in sandwiches and casseroles, omelets, pizzas, and stir-fries. Eat a handful of parsley or fennel after a meal to sweeten your breath and give you concentrated vitamins and minerals. Try a new vegetable or fruit every week.

Nutrient-Dense Foods Add blackstrap molasses, broccoli, dandelion greens, kelp, salmon with bones, sardines, mackerel, nuts, and seeds to your diet to reduce inflammation and add needed minerals. Don't be afraid to eat nuts: 1 ounce of walnuts or almonds adds only 164 calories but can keep you satisfied so that you don't overeat.

Tryptophan-Rich Foods Tryptophan aids in weight loss by reducing appetite. Eat more foods that contain this essential amino acid.

Foods rich in tryptophan include brown rice, cottage cheese, turkey, peanuts, and soy protein.

Whole Grains and Legumes   Eat more whole grains (brown rice, whole wheat, bulgur, millet, buckwheat, rye, barley, spelt, oats, quinoa) and legumes (dried beans, dried peas, lentils, peanuts). Studies show the fiber protects your colon, reduces risk of colon and breast cancer, and fills you up so you don't overeat.

Herbs

Emma had her own parenting class business. She was 50 and a widowed grandmother. She carved out a space for herself as an independent woman, making a good income and traveling around the country giving workshops. When menopause changes began, she felt unprepared and unsure. Emma suffered from intense hot flashes that kept her from sleeping. She'd tried nutritional approaches, but none helped. When she came to see me, she told me that a friend had been raving about how much herbs had helped. Emma wanted to know the advantages and disadvantages of taking herbs and whether she should take them.

You may have heard about using herbs for menopause symptoms but may not be sure which herbs to take and which to avoid. This chapter provides information to help you decide.

Every culture has at some point used healing plants as the basis for its healing procedures. Herbal remedies are found with the Indian Ayurvedic, Chinese, and Native American healing systems. Herbs have been used for thousands of years and their safety in many situations has been established. Until 50 years ago, nearly all entries in the medical pharmacopoeias described treatments of an herbal origin. These entries were based on numerous published studies on the effects of herbs on animal and human physiology. When modern drug companies launched their synthetic products, they could be patented for profit, so medical botany and the masters who historically handed down the art and science of herbology were abandoned in the United States. The Europeans and Chinese have never abandoned their herbal roots. They have been conducting research for a long time, and the German E Commission, the authority on research-backed herb research, has developed principles of herb application. Practitioners in the United States are starting to acknowledge this alternative/complementary approach to health.

Unlike modern medicine, herbal science recognizes the body as a whole, integrated system greater than the sum of its parts. Ancient cultures were aware of the organizing power of nature, a unified or bioenergy field that exists at the deepest level. This dynamic energy field is a life-promoting force within and around plants and humans that nourishes and fortifies. As part of the natural order of things, plants restore human chemistry by targeting specific receptors within the body, bringing health and balance. Herbs are much more difficult to misuse than drugs because their active ingredients are diluted by plant material, act more slowly than medicines, and are used primarily to mobilize self-healing capabilities, working at deeper levels than synthetic medicines, which are targeted at symptoms.

Herbs are potent substances that don't work well with many medicines. Always talk to your health care provider about the herbs you plan to take or are taking so that your care can be coordinated. Never take herbs when pregnant, for longer than is recommended, or in higher than suggested doses.

■ Breast Cancer and Other Cancers

Focus On:

Black Cohosh   According to *Clinician Reviews*, black cohosh is an herb from the buttercup family. The herb exerts its effects on the endocrine regulatory (hormonal) mechanism in your body. It's a phytoestrogen, meaning it's weaker than the estrogens your body creates. Structurally, black cohosh more closely resembles estriol, which researchers believe offers protection against cancer of the endometrium, ovaries, and breast. You can take black cohosh for menopausal symptoms, and you may get protection against cancer at the same time.

Lemon Balm   Lemon balm oil was shown to be effective against a series of human cancer cell lines. These results point to the potential use of lemon balm as an antitumor agent.

Licorice Root   Laboratory fractionations of extracts of licorice root were used to determine its ability to inhibit cell proliferation in human breast cancer cells. The researchers concluded that licorice root may have chemopreventive effects against breast cancer.

Red Clover   Dozens of studies show that phytoestrogens like red clover inhibit the growth of breast cancer cells. One study presented evidence that red clover in a supplement called Promensil reduced breast tissue density in postmenopausal women. This is encouraging, since an increase in density is associated with a higher risk of breast cancer.

■ Cold Hands

Focus On:

Stimulants   Cayenne pepper, ginkgo, and ginger are all circulatory stimulants that could increase circulation.

Tonics   If cold hands are due to thyroid inefficiency, tonic herbs such as astragalus root may be helpful. Astragalus can be taken as a tea or in capsules.

■ Depression, Nervousness, and Irritability

Focus On:

Ashwagandha This Indian herb has been shown to stabilize mood and reduce depression. It appears to be safe but hasn't been studied extensively.

Black Cohosh Consider black cohosh, especially if depression is due to natural or surgically induced menopause. See the Hot Flashes section for more information about this herb.

St. John's-Wort and Ginkgo Biloba Based on available research, the *German Commission E Monographs* (considered the authority on herb research) recommend 900 mg/day of St. John's-wort in divided doses of a 0.3% standardized product and 120–240 mg native dry extract of ginkgo biloba in two or three doses.

■ Dizziness

Focus On:

Black Cohosh In a study of 704 women, 49% who took a black cohosh preparation experienced complete relief of menopausal symptoms including vertigo or dizziness. An additional 37.8% reported significant improvement. According to the physicians who conducted the study, 72% of the women who took the black cohosh treatment experienced advantages over those given hormonal treatment (as measured by results on the Kupperman Menopausal Index and the Hamilton Anxiety Test).

Gingko Biloba Based on available research, the *German Commission E Monographs* recommend 120–240 mg/day of ginkgo biloba native dry extract in two or three doses.

■ Fatigue

Focus On:

Ginseng Based on available research, the *German Commission E Monographs* recommend 1–2 grams of ginseng root a day to reduce fatigue and increase energy.

■ Hair Loss/Thinning

Focus On:

Horsetail and Oat Straw The herbs horsetail and oat straw are both rich in silica, which is necessary for strong, shiny hair.

Herbs That Contain B-Vitamins Herbs that contain B-vitamins, so important for hair health, include cayenne, chamomile, eyebright, fennel, fenugreek, nettle, oat straw, parsley, peppermint, raspberry leaf, red clover, and catnip.

Herbs That Contain Vitamin C Herbs that contain vitamin C include cayenne, chickweed, eyebright, fennel seed, fenugreek, horsetail, peppermint, nettle, oat straw, paprika, parsley, raspberry leaf, red clover, rose hips, and skullcap.

Herbs That Contain Vitamin E Herbs that contain vitamin E include dandelion, flaxseed, nettle, oat straw, raspberry leaf, and rose hips.

Herbs That Contain Zinc Herbs that contain zinc include chamomile, eyebright, fennel seed, milk thistle, nettle, parsley, skullcap, and wild yam.

■ Headaches

Focus On:

Black Cohosh In a study of 704 women, 49% who took a black cohosh preparation experienced complete relief of menopausal symptoms including headache. An additional 37.8% reported significant improvement. According to the physicians who conducted the study, 72% of the women who took the black cohosh treatment experienced advantages over those given hormonal treatment (as measured by results on the Kupperman Menopausal Index and the Hamilton Anxiety Test).

Butterbur Two ingredients in butterbur inhibit the production of *leukotrienes*, which are compounds that trigger inflammation of blood vessels. Headaches occur when cerebral blood vessels contract and then expand, stimulating pain receptors. Several studies have shown that butterbur can reduce headaches by 34% to 50%. The dose is a 50 mg capsule two to three times a day. It takes up to 1 month to see benefits; the best results are seen after 4–6 months, and you should stop taking the herb at this point. (You can resume taking butterbur for another 4–6 months if headaches recur.) The only possible side effect is occasional stomach upset. Only the capsules with the pyrrolizidine alkaloids (Pas) removed or with a daily maximum dose of no more than 1 mcg of Pas should be taken, as Pas are toxic and can damage the liver. Consult with your health care provider before taking butterbur if you are pregnant, nursing, or if you have liver or kidney disease.

Chasteberry According to the National Women's Health Center, chasteberry, also known as monk's pepper, Indian spice, sage tree hemp, or tree wild pepper, has been found to help women with headache symptoms.

Phytoestrogen Supplements One study of 49 women showed that those who received a phytoestrogen preparation consisting of 60 mg soy isoflavones, 100 mg dong quai, and 50 mg black cohosh reduced their migraine attacks by more than half compared with women taking a placebo (sugar pill).

St. John's-Wort Based on available research, the *German Commission E Monographs* recommend 900 mg/day of St. John's-wort in divided doses of a 0.3% standardized product and 120–240 mg native dry extract of ginkgo biloba in two or three doses.

White Willow White willow is approved by the German Commission E for headache.

■ Heart and Blood Vessel Disease

Focus On:

Ashwagandha Studies indicate ashwagandha exerts a positive effect on the heart and lungs and appears to be safe.

Black Cohosh In a study of 704 women, 49% who took the black cohosh preparation experienced complete relief of menopausal symptoms (hot flashes, sweating, headache, vertigo, heart palpitations, and ringing in the ears.) An additional 37.8% reported significant improvement. According to the physicians who conducted the study, 72% of the women who took the black cohosh treatment experienced advantages over those given hormonal treatment (as measured by results on the Kupperman Menopausal Index and the Hamilton Anxiety Test).

Dandi Tablet In a study of 73 postmenopausal women, half were given an herbal supplement called Dandi Tablet, and the other half were given nylestriol. The Dandi group showed elevated levels of estrogen and improved blood fats. The researchers concluded the Dandi Tablet showed a heart disease–preventive effect.

Red Clover Fifty milligrams of red clover have been shown to help cholesterol by raising the level of the good HDL. This means better heart protection. In another study, women who received 80 mg of isoflavones from red clover improved the elasticity of their arteries by 23%. More pliable blood vessels protects you from developing heart disease.

■ Hot Flashes

Focus On:

Black Cohosh This herb does not promote breast cancer cell growth as once thought, but it does reduce hot flashes, adverse effects are extremely uncommon, and there are no known significant adverse drug interactions. A daily dose of 40 mg of the root extract effectively treats symptoms. Find a standardized product such as Remifemin (20 mg twice a day). You can expect to see improvement in 4–8 weeks of use. Most experts suggest that you take a break from the herb after 6 months because the effect of long-term use has not been studied.

Do not use black cohosh if you are taking medication for high blood pressure or if you are pregnant, except under the supervision of a health care practitioner. Discontinue use if you experience any new symptoms after beginning to use the herb.

In a study of 704 women, 49% who took the preparation experienced complete relief of menopausal symptoms including hot flashes. An additional 37.8% reported significant improvement. According to the physicians who conducted the study, 72% of the women who took the black cohosh treatment experienced advantages over those given hormonal treatment (as measured by results on the Kupperman Menopausal Index and the Hamilton Anxiety Test). In another controlled study of 629 women with menopausal complaints who took a standardized extract of black cohosh twice a day, 76% to 93% had an overall improvement in hot flashes, headache, irritability, heart palpitations, mild depression, and sleep disturbances. The reduction in headache, sleep disturbances, and heart palpitations is understandable because black cohosh also contains a small amount of salicylic acid (used to make aspirin) that has anti-inflammatory and pain-relieving qualities. But black cohosh has also been proven to help women who have undergone hysterectomy with partial removal of their ovaries.

How safe is this herb? More than 40 years of use in Germany has shown no evidence of serious adverse effects, contraindications, or drug interactions. The only side effect appeared in just 7% of the participants in one of many studies. In this case, the women experienced a short-term stomach upset but not enough to stop taking the herb, and the problem didn't continue for long.

Another study critically evaluated the safety of black cohosh. The researchers examined all published studies, the FDA and World Health Organization adverse-event reporting systems, monographs, data from major manufacturers, and anecdotal reports. Human trials of more than 2,800 women demonstrated a very low incidence of adverse events (5.4%). Of these, 97% were minor and the only severe events were not attributed to taking black cohosh at all.

An important consideration for long-term use of black cohosh or any substance is its potential toxicity and cancer-causing attributes. Researchers at Northwestern Medical School found that black cohosh extracts do not demonstrate any estrogenic activity (associated with breast cancer), so in that respect black cohosh is safe. An alarm was sounded in the summer of 2003 in an Australian case report, but the findings were not sufficiently substantiated; also, a case report of one person's reactions does not provide strong evidence compared with human trials of thousands of women.

So far, no overdose amount has been found for black cohosh in humans. In one study involving animals given 90 times the daily human equivalent, no negative results were found.

The research shows that for the majority of menopausal women taking black cohosh, it is safe and effective, but if you are experiencing heavy menstrual bleeding, black cohosh may increase it. If you have a negative reaction, stop taking the herb and consult with your health care practitioner. (If you have liver disease or are pregnant, this is not a herb for you.) In any event, it's always a good idea to talk to your health care practitioners about herbs you are taking or planning to take and why, to make sure they do not negatively interact with any drugs (either prescribed or over-the-counter) you may be taking.

A study conducted by Enzymatic Therapy, a producer of herbal formulas, focused on the efficacy of a morning/evening menopause formula (morning capsule contains panax ginseng, black cohosh, soy, and green tea extracts; evening capsule contains black cohosh, soy, kava, hops, and valerian extracts) for relieving hot flashes. The combined formula significantly reduced the number of hot flashes reported by healthy postmenopausal women between 45 and 65 years of age. A 47% reduction of hot flashes was observed as early as the end of the second week.

Red Clover   Several studies have provided evidence that red clover helps some women. If you are taking blood thinners or anticoagulants, don't take red clover because it contains its own blood thinners. Red clover can be found in health food or herb stores as a tea, capsule, or tincture. You may even find red clover in your backyard. According to Tammi Hartung, a medical herbalist, two 500 mg capsules are taken three times a day with meals, but it may take 3–6 weeks to see results. For tea, 1–3 teaspoons of dried red clover are added to a cup of boiling water and allowed to steep for 10–15 minutes. Drink a cup 3 times a day.

Sage and Alfalfa   One study examined the effect of a plant product based on extracts of the leaves of sage and alfalfa in 30 menopausal women. Hot flashes completely disappeared in 20 women, 4 women showed good improvement, and the other 6 showed some reduction in symptoms. No side effects were noted.

■ Insomnia/Sleep Problems

Focus On:

Chamomile Chamomile is a mild herb that can safely be used unless you're allergic to flowers or ragweed. It can relax you and prepare you for sleep. Simply put a tea bag in a cup and fill with hot water. Let it steep a few minutes and enjoy its sweet, pleasant flavor.

Herbal Combination Capsule Use a morning/evening menopause formula from Enzymatic Therapy (morning capsule contains panax ginseng, black cohosh, soy, and green tea extracts; evening capsule contains black cohosh, soy, kava, hops, and valerian extracts) for relieving menopausal symptoms such as sleep disturbance. The combined formula significantly increases sleep quality.

Kava Kava is a much stronger herb than chamomile. It has been used in a multicenter, randomized, double-blind clinical study. Results after 4 weeks showed quality of sleep and recuperative effect after sleep were significantly superior to a placebo. Safety and tolerability were good, with no adverse events or changes. The researchers concluded that sleep disturbances associated with non-psychotic anxiety can be effectively and safely treated with 200 mg kava extract. (Although there have been reports in newspapers about kava damaging the liver, two-thirds of the 30 cases reported involved abuse of drugs and/or alcohol, both of which can also damage the liver, as can the over-the-counter pain medication Tylenol).

According to Hyla Cass, MD, kava should not be used by anyone who has liver problems or by anyone who is taking drug products with known adverse effects on the liver, is a regular consumer of alcohol, or who has symptoms of jaundice (e.g., dark urine, yellowing of the eyes). Kava should not be taken for more than 3 months, which is the German Commission E's recommendation. The maximum daily intake should not exceed 250 mg kavalactones (2 tablets or capsules) or 3 g of dried rhizome per tea bag.

Lemon Balm Lemon balm has been widely used as a mild sedative.

Melatonin Melatonin reduces the time it takes to fall asleep and nighttime awakenings. As a result, you may feel more alert the next day after taking it. While most studies indicate that melatonin is safe, its long-term effects and ideal dosage are still in question. Studies have shown melatonin to work in amounts ranging from 0.1 mg to 5 mg taken 30 minutes before bedtime.

Valerian Valerian has been shown to improve sleep quality after 600 mg of the extract were taken, and found as effective as the drug oxazepam. Results of taking single doses of the herb are contradictory. While the adverse effect profile and tolerability of this herb are excellent, long-term safety studies are lacking. Valerian doesn't appear to have a detrimental effect on thinking or movement performance at a dose of 500 mg or 1,000 mg. The herb may potentiate the effects of anesthetics, so it is wise not to take valerian for a week prior to having anesthesia.

■ Itchiness

Focus On:

Black Cohosh You may want to consider taking black cohosh if you have itchiness due to natural or surgically-induced menopause. See Hot Flashes section for more information.

Chamomile Flower extracts of German chamomile worked as well as oxatomide, an antiallergic agent, in a study of mice induced to scratching behavior. If you're not allergic to flowers or ragweed, chamomile should be safe for you to try.

■ Joint and Muscle Pain

Focus On:

Nettle Research has shown that a water extract of nettle has an analgesic and pain reduction effect.

White Willow White willow contains salicin, a form of salicylate, which is closely related to modern aspirin (acetylsalicylic acid). It is known to the Greeks for its medicinal uses against fever and pain, and approved by the German Commission E as a remedy for pain and rheumatism. Side effects may include indigestion, nausea, and ringing in the ears. White willow was listed in the U.S. pharmacopoeias from 1820 to 1880.

■ Memory Loss and Foggy Thinking

Focus On:

Gingko Biloba A review of studies of age-associated memory impairment treated with 120–240 mg native dry gingko biloba extract reveals that it has positive effects on thinking functions and is well tolerated.

Lemon Balm Lemon balm improves memory performance and increases calmness when the encapsulated dried leaf is taken at 600, 1,000, or 1,600 mg, at 7-day intervals. In one study the greatest improvement was at the highest dose.

Licorice Root An animal study showed that licorice root (glycyrrhiza, not the candy) enhanced memory. The antiinflammatory and antioxidant properties of licorice may be what contributes favorably to memory enhancement. Licorice is known to raise blood pressure and should be used with caution in those with high blood pressure.

St. John's-Wort Based on available research, the *German Commission E Monographs* recommend 900 mg/day of St. John's-wort in divided doses of a 0.3% standardized product.

■ Menstrual Bleeding

Three herbs may be especially helpful for excessive bleeding.

Focus On:

Red Raspberry The red raspberry leaf is an astringent that promotes drying. It's milder than shepherd's purse, so it could take up to 3 ounces daily brewed as a tea to slow menstrual flow.

Shepherd's Purse Shepherd's purse leaf tea has a long history as a remedy for menstrual bleeding. Use 0.25 to 0.5 ounces brewed as a tea. Although it tastes terrible, it can work in hours or even minutes, so you'll probably only need one cup for each incidence of bleeding.

Turmeric Turmeric can stop bleeding. Taken in capsules, use as a spice on food, or mix into a paste.

■ Osteoporosis

Focus On:

Black Cohosh Results of animal studies in Japan suggest that one variety of black cohosh may increase bone mineral density.

Puerariae Radix Puerariae radix (PR), the root of a wild creeper leguminous plant, is one of the earliest and most important crude herbs used in Chinese medicine. PR contains a high amount of isoflavonoids such as daidzein and genistein, which are known to prevent bone loss induced by low estrogen levels. In a study with mice that had their ovaries removed, PR completely prevented a decrease in bone density and restored bone thickness. The researchers concluded PR may be an alternative treatment in the prevention of osteoporosis in postmenopausal women.

Red Clover Red clover has been shown to reduce bone loss in healthy women. Although it contains phytoestrogens, it does not cause an increase in breast density, so it is unlikely to increase breast cancer risk.

■ Sex Drive Reduction or Intercourse Discomfort

Focus On:

Angelica Also known as dong quai, this herb is often referred to as the "female ginseng." It is believed to have a balancing effect on the female hormonal system and act as an all-purpose sexual and reproductive tonic. The dosage is 3 to 4 grams a day. Avoid if pregnant or experiencing heavy menstrual bleeding.

Black Cohosh Consider this herb if you have vaginal pain or itching due to natural or surgically induced menopause. Don't use if experiencing heavy menstrual bleeding. See the Hot Flashes section for more information.

Damiana According to Dr. Sarah Brewer, damiana shows promise as a sexual desire booster. The Maya in Central America have used damiana as a traditional aphrodisiac. It contains alkaloids that may boost circulation to the genital area and increase nerve endings sensitivity in the clitoris and penis. Damiana is said to increase sexual desire, stimulate sexual performance, and enhance pleasure. One to two 400 mg capsules taken on an occasional basis is the dose recommended by Dr. Brewer. She says there are no cautions and it can be combined with ginseng.

Gingko Biloba Gingko biloba, one of the oldest known plants on Earth, improves circulation and could enhance sexual desire. It boots circulation to the hands, feet, and brain. Research suggests it may improve blood flow to the genitals even at a low dose of 60 mg daily. It may not take effect for up to 10 days, but once reached, the effects last for 3–6 hours.

Ginseng In the article "Sex Treatment," Dr. Sarah Brewer suggests taking Korean ginseng, an herb that has been used in China as a sexual balancer and revitalizer for thousands of years and in India as an aphrodisiac. Clinical studies have confirmed ginseng has a normalizing effect on hormone imbalances, improves peripheral blood flow (including to the genitals), and helps the body adjust to stress and fatigue. Ginseng should not be taken for more than 6 weeks without a break. Dr. Brewer suggests 200–1,000 mg/day on a 2-week-on, 2-week-off cycle. Avoid if you have high blood pressure, glaucoma, or breast cancer.

Oat Extract The unripe oat grain is used as an antidepressant and as a restorative nerve tonic to relieve stress and exhaustion. If this is your source of low sexual desire, consider taking the oat extract or tincture. Follow the directions on the bottle. If you're sensitive to gluten (celiac disease), only take the tincture after allowing it to settle and scooping off the clear liquid for use.

St. John's-Wort If depression or exhaustion is lowering your sexual desire, St. John's-wort (hypericum) may help. This herb has been used for thousands of years to enhance emotional well-being. Since low sex drive and lack of desire can be an early feature of depression, hypericum may be especially helpful if depression is the problem.

Researchers in Germany tested 111 postmenopausal women and found of those taking hypericum who were physically exhausted and had low sex drive, 60% developed an interest in sex again, felt sexy, and enjoyed or even initiated sex. Hypericum also helped 82% reduce anxiety, depression, hot flashes, sweating, and disturbed sleep.

The good thing about hypericum is that it can even be used with estrogen replacement therapy. Dr. Brewer recommends 300 mg three times a day. Stay out of strong sunlight or cover your body well and wear a hat. Hypericum can cause dermatitis if skin is exposed to sunlight.

Vitex Also called chasteberry, vitex corrects hormonal imbalances, including sexual imbalance. It is a gentle herb and may take several months to show results and up to a year to see permanent changes when you can stop taking the herb. The usual dosage is 40 drops in a glass of water in the morning. It should never be used when pregnant.

■ Skin Problems

Focus On:

Gotu Kola Gota kola improves the integrity and function of connective tissue, increase blood supply to tissues, and helps form healthy skin. Drink it as a tea or pat on your skin. One to two ounces of the herb per day is used for acute conditions. As a long-term tonic, 1 to 2 capsules is appropriate.

■ Urinary Symptoms

Focus On:

Cornsilk This herb can reduce bladder spasms and has a diuretic effect. It's usually available in capsules or as a tea. Follow directions on the label.

Nettle Nettle has long been used to treat urinary problems. A study has shown its antimicrobial activity against nine microorganisms, so it may be beneficial for bladder infections as well as to enhance urinary function.

■ Weight Gain

Focus On:

Licorice Licorice the herb, not the candy, reduced body fat in adults who consumed 3.5 grams a day of a commercial preparation for 2 months. Researchers concluded that licorice can reduce body fat. (Use the deglycyrrhizinated licorice root [DGL] so that there is no risk of raising blood pressure regardless of dosage.)

Environmental Actions

There are many things you can do to create a healthy and supportive environment during and after menopause. This chapter describes some of the most effective and well-known ones as well as things to avoid.

■ Breast Cancer and Other Cancers

Avoid:

Xenoestrogens Chemicals in your environment can mimic estrogen, increasing your risk of breast cancer. Protect yourself by not using pesticides or drinking tap water, avoiding freshwater fish that contain PCBs and DDT, and losing weight if you need to (pollutants are fat-soluble and concentrate in fatty tissue such as breasts).

Radiation Because of potential low-level radiation leakage, avoid microwave ovens. Do not sit close to television sets; sit at least eight feet away. Avoid X-rays.

Other Suspected Carcinogens Chemicals such as hairsprays, cleaning compounds, waxes, fresh paints, pesticides, art and craft supplies, cosmetics, varnishes, carpet glues, drugs (unless prescribed).

Focus On:

Non-Polluted Substances Drink distilled water or purchase a reverse osmosis filtration system to ensure the purest possible water. Buy a shower filter to decrease the chance of pollutants entering through your skin. Make sure you ingest the fewest pollutants by eating the kinds of seafood least likely to be polluted: shrimp, chunk light tuna, haddock, cod, fish stick, tilapia, and pollock. Purchase organically grown produce that is not grown with herbicides or pesticides. Eat only meat that has not been produced with hormones and antibiotics. Eat only poultry that has grown up in a free ranging environment.

■ Cold Hands

Avoid:

Stressful Environments Stay away from cold and stressful environments; they can result in cold extremities. Avoid drinking water that contains fluoride and chlorine; they block iodine receptors in the thyroid gland and can lead to hypothyroidism, a symptom of which is cold hands.

Focus On:

Ginger Compresses Use ginger compresses to relax muscle tension and promote circulation to the hands, thereby warming them. Place a golf ball size of fresh grated ginger root in cheesecloth or a handkerchief and dip in 3–4 quarts of water that has just been boiled and taken off the burner. When the water is still hot but not burning, wring the cloth out and place on your hands. Place a dry towel on top or ask a family member to help. Apply a fresh hot towel every minute or so until the skin becomes red, about 15–20 minutes.

Keeping Warm Keep a pair of gloves handy and put them on to keep your hands warm.

Massage Massage your hands several times a day to enhance circulation.

■ Depression, Nervousness, and Irritability

Lack of direction and purpose as well as unresolved losses can lead to depression.

Avoid:

Depression-Evoking Situations Don't smoke, take steroids, anti-depressants or oral contraceptives. All have been associated with depression. Avoid negative thinking and being unprepared for work, school, or other obligations.

Focus On:

Volunteering Volunteering to help others is a great way to overcome depression. If you're feeling too depressed to take action, call a counselor to help you.

■ Dizziness

Avoid:

Activities That Bring on Dizziness Some activities that can bring on dizziness include amusement park rides, action movies, playing virtual reality games, riding in the back seat of a car, and riding in a boat.

Focus On:

Moving Slowly Refrain from standing too quickly or sitting up quickly from a lying position.

■ Fatigue

Avoid:

Situations That Evoke Fatigue Missing sleep and overdoing can stress and fatigue you.

Focus On:

Time and Activity Management Plan your activities so you don't have to go back and forth to get items or complete tasks. Don't overschedule yourself. If you're not sure what to do, buy a good book on the subject or take a time management course.

■ Hair Loss/Thinning

Avoid:

Styling Methods That Damage Hair Using a hair dryer, combing your hair when it's wet, and brushing your hair too much can damage it.

Focus On:

Safe Hair Handling Let your hair air dry and comb your hair with a hair pick.

■ Headaches

Avoid:

Phthalates Phthhalates are plasticizers. You can identify them indoors by that new plastic smell. Get rid of plastics and replace them with natural materials whenever possible.

Focus On:

Using Natural Materials Replace plastics with natural materials such as cotton, glass, paper, or wood. Purchase sisal or wool carpets from Naturlich at nathome@monitor.net. Purchase environmentally sound furniture from Furnature at furnature@tiac.net.

■ Heart Disease

Avoid:

Smoking Smoking increases your risk of heart conditions.

Focus On:

Making Your Environment Healthier Stop smoking if you smoke and arrange your living environment for low stress.

■ Hot Flashes

Avoid:

Warming Environments

Focus On:

Using a Cooling Mist Look for Emerita's Cooling Comfort Mist, a spritzer containing witch hazel, peppermint, menthol, and lemon.

Spritz on at first flush. Keep it beside you and on your nightstand for a cool-off.

Fans   Experiment with hand fans and small electric or battery-operated fans as a way to cool off and relax. Keep a hand fan on your bedside table and grab it when a hot flash wakes you up. Carry a fan and a thermos of cool water for relief.

Layering Clothes   Wear 2–4 layers of clothes. Remove top layers during hot flashes.

Peppermint Essential Oil   Add a couple of drops of peppermint essential oil to castor oil, olive oil, or a natural body lotion. You can find essential oils at your health food store. The peppermint has a cooling effect. Be sure not to get it anywhere near your eyes, and wash your hands after putting it on your arms, neck, chest, buttocks, legs, and feet. If you don't feel anything, add another drop or two, then wait for the cooling effect. It will last about half an hour.

■ Insomnia/Sleep Problems

Avoid:

Antidepressants   Most antidepressants interfere with sleep. Find alternate approaches to your depression. (See chapters 4–9 for ideas.)

Caffeine   Caffeine is a great sleep robber. Once you get off caffeine, you'll be perkier and more grounded. You won't need the ups and downs that caffeine gives you. Start slowly by using half caffeinated coffee and half decaffeinated coffee. Slowly increase the decaffeinated coffee until you are drinking it 100%.

Cigarette Smoke   The chemicals in cigarette smoke can keep you awake. Take a smoking cessation course with your local Lung Association or have your family agree to smoke only outside until you can convince them to stop smoking.

Eating When Unable to Sleep   When your body is trying to digest food, it is more difficult to sleep. Use stress reduction measures if something is bothering you (see chapter 8).

Late Evening Meals and Strenuous Exercise   Overloading your body with food and your mind with stimulation is a recipe for staying awake.

Focus On:

Eating an Early and Light Dinner   You don't want to be digesting food when you're trying to sleep. Your body needs at least 3 hours after a meal for digestion.

Good Sleep Habits   Only use the bed for sleep and sex. If you're not sleeping after lying quietly for 10 minutes, get up and engage in some relaxing activity.

Keeping a Sleep Log   Write down pertinent events (heavy meals, exercise, stress), hot flash occurrences, caffeine and alcohol use, and so on. Chart the pattern of what keeps you awake and then take action.

Calming Music   Not just any music will bring on sleep. It must have a largo beat (60 beats a minute or less) found in compositions by Bach, Handel, Vivaldi, and Corelli. Record the largo or adaggio movements from their baroque compositions and play them before bedtime.

Therapeutic Baths   Experiment with therapeutic baths that can soothe you from stress and overworking (or overplaying) and calm you down so you can sleep. Throw in a capful of lavender, chamomile, or patchouli essential oil and enjoy.

■ Itchiness

Avoid:

Harmful Chemicals   Don't use cleaners, lotions, waxes, disinfectants, or other products that contain harmful chemicals, fragrances or perservatives including organochlorine pesticides, chlorine, phenols used in furniture polish, wood preservatives, acetone, benzene, naptha, toluene, xylene, ethanes, ethylenes, ketones, ammonia, formaldehyde and polymer resins. Launder bedding and other fabrics only with non-allergenic soap. Avoid deodorizers and disinfectants; their main purpose is to mask odors, not clean.

Focus On:

Soothing Lotions Find a good lotion without synthetic chemicals, fragrances, or preservatives to use on all skin surfaces. Aubrey makes products with 100% natural ingredients (www.aubrey-organics.com). Try castor oil, aloe vera gel, jojoba oil, or olive oil to see which works best on your skin. These products can also be inserted in the vagina to stop itching.

Safe Cleaners Use baking soda, borax, vinegar, non-chlorine bleach, mineral oil, or beeswax.

■ Joint and Muscle Pain

Avoid:

Extremes Stay away from extreme temperatures, overdoing, stressing or straining muscles or joints, or being overweight (can aggravate joint stress).

Focus On:

Muscle Balms White Flower Analgesic Balm is a rub-on liquid and Tiger Balm is a salve. Both warm the affected area and bring healing nutrients via your circulation to your aching muscles. Both can be found at your local health food store.

Therapeutic Baths Find Dr. Singha's Mustard Bath, ABRA Herbal Hydrotherapy Baths, or Therapeutic Bath Herbs at your local health food or herb store. Follow the directions and let yourself heal.

■ Memory Loss and Foggy Thinking

Avoid:

Multitasking Doing too much at one time impairs your memory. Switching between complex tasks can slow you down by 25% to 50%

Specific Drugs Cough suppressants, some pain relievers, prednisone, sleep aids, and antidiarrheal drugs are common brain foggers. Avoid them and find a natural alternative.

Tobacco and Alcohol Both alcohol and tobacco sap your brain of its quick wit and sharp focus. Avoid them, including secondhand smoke.

Toxins Steer clear of toxics, including heavy metals such as lead and mercury. They are well known for dimming memory. So are fluoride (fluoridated water and toothpaste) and aluminum (in pots, water, food, and drugs).

Focus On:

Arranging Information Try word association games to help you with names and other important information.

Identifying Core Intentions Instead of focusing on three things at once, ask, "What three things can I focus on today that will lead me to fulfilling my core intentions for the week?"

Setting Realistic Goals Instead of underestimating how long something will actually take and overcommitting, schedule one less thing than you think you can do and enjoy a long lunch or a pleasant break.

Taking Breaks Set a timer and make sure you take a break at least every 90 minutes. Let your brain recharge!

Delegating More Identify what you can delegate and do it. Start small with a holiday or birthday. Let the store wrap the presents. Instead of baking cookies to bring to school or a party, buy them. Ask for help from your spouse, partner, kids, or friends. (Be sure to repay whoever helps you out!)

Learning to Say No   Think of saying no as a creative act. It will give you a chance to be more present with what you've agreed to.

Cleaning Off Your Desk   You can focus more easily when you clean off your desk.

Giving Up Being Perfect   Excellence is a wonderful quality; perfectionism is dangerous. Do your best and let it be.

Subliminal Stimulation   Short-term recall can be enhanced by listening to subliminal presentations of memory improvement affirmations embedded in relaxing music. If you want to better your memory, you can obtain this type of tape from Louise Hay, who pioneered the use of affirmation and metaphysical self-healing approaches. Call her at (800)-654-5126 or visit her Web site at http://www.hayhouse.com.

■ Menstrual Bleeding

Avoid:

Smoking   If you smoke, you're at a higher risk for abnormal vaginal bleeding.

Focus On:

Quitting Smoking   Refer to the Osteoporosis section for suggestions.

Castor Oil Packs   Castor oil packs have provided effective relief for countless women suffering from heavy menstrual bleeding no matter what the cause. Heritage Products at www.caycecures.com offers organic castor oil and directions on castor oil packs.

■ Osteoporosis

Avoid:

Mineral-Leaching Drugs   Many drugs leach minerals, including calcium, from your body. Check with package inserts and/or a good reference such as Mindell and Hopkins's *Prescription Alternatives* to find out if you are taking any prescribed or over-the-counter drugs that may lead to osteoporosis.

Quitting Smoking   Smoking is associated with osteoporosis.

> *Elizabeth had been smoking for forty years. She ran her own pet shop and had written several books on the selection and care of pets. Cigarettes were her constant companion while she wrote and on her work breaks. Her father had died of lung cancer, and Elizabeth had already been diagnosed with emphysema. She feared she might develop cancer herself. Elizabeth had tried to stop smoking several times in the past and had temporarily succeeded twice, but each time she had returned to smoking under stress. When she came to see me, she was convinced she was ready to stop smoking for good. She joined one of my smoking cessation groups, found a buddy to provide support between sessions, and started a walking program. It took her 6 months, but eventually she was able to quit smoking.*

Focus On:

If you haven't quit, now's the time. You can be just as successful as Elizabeth. (If people in your household smoke, that puts you at risk for osteoporosis. Try to convince them to quit. If you can't, insist that they smoke outside the house only.)

Here are some tips for quitting smoking you (or your family member) can use:

1. Ask yourself, "What is this habit doing for me?" (It's doing something or you wouldn't keep it!)

2. Ask yourself, "What is this habit costing me?"

3. Decide how you could get these things without using so much negative energy.

4. Write your plan for what you will start to do today to quit smoking. (Join a group and find a supportive buddy to work along with you.)

5. Eat more fruits, vegetables, and grains. Eat half a grapefruit after a meal to reduce the urge to smoke, then brush your teeth.

6. Avoid caffeinated drinks, which increase cravings for cigarettes. Avoid alcohol because it decreases your willpower.

7. Drink 8 glasses of water a day and avoid drinks with a lot of calories—sodas, juices, and milk—that can add weight.

8. Get rid of all cigarettes and ashtrays in your home, car, and workplace.

9. Ask your family, friends, and coworkers for support.

10. Stay in nonsmoking areas.

11. Breathe in and out deeply and wait 5 minutes (by the clock) when you feel the urge to smoke (second month, increase the wait to 10 minutes, third month, increase it to 15 minutes).

12. Keep yourself busy. Hold something other than a cigarette in your hand—for example, cinnamon stick, toothpick, pen or pencil, straw. Take up a hobby that occupies your hands—for example, knitting, crocheting, painting, playing an instrument, writing. Cut up raw vegetables and have one or chew a piece of gum when you have an urge to smoke.

13. Reward yourself often, especially by planning a present for yourself with the money you save from not smoking.

14. Set a quit date (in writing) and stick to it. Quitting cold turkey is best and is associated with the fewest with-

drawal symptoms. (Physical addiction to nicotine only lasts for 48 hours—you can do it!)

15. Learn relaxation skills (see chapter 8).

16. Do at least one enjoyable activity every day.

17. Remind yourself of the rewards of quitting: improved health, food will taste better, improved sense of smell, save money, feel better about yourself, home/car/breath will smell better, can stop worrying about quitting, set a good example for others, no worries about exposing others to smoke, feel better physically, freedom from addiction, perform better at sports, less chance of cancer and other illnesses.

18. Start an exercise program and follow it.

■ Sex Drive Reduction or Intercourse Discomfort

Avoid:

Drugs That Reduce Sex Drive/Orgasms Antidepressants are known to reduce interest in sex and ability to perform. Check every drug you take for sex-drive effects with a *Physicians' Desk Reference* (PDR) online or at your library reference desk.

Feminine Products The following products can interfere with orgasm and sexual function by causing irritation and itching: perfumed soap, feminine hygiene sprays, bubble baths, packaged douches (your vagina cleans itself; douches only destroy the pH balance and set you up for an infection), panty hose and panties without cotton crotches, antihistamines (which can dry the mucous membranes in your vagina).

Focus On:

Touching and Kissing More Ban the quick peck on the check or lips. Go for long, deep, sensuous kisses several times a day. Ask your partner for hugs many times a day. Hold hands and watch the sunset or go for a walk after dinner. Don't forget the sensuousness of massage. Use a scented oil and massage each other as a prelude to intercourse.

Wearing Something Sexy Find an outfit that makes you feel attractive and that your partner likes. You can ask in advance, perhaps showing several outfits and asking for feedback.

Changing Location Talk to your partner about going away for a weekend or making love in the living room instead of the bedroom. Discuss various alternatives.

Lubricating Your Vagina Prick several vitamin E capsules with a pin and squeeze the oil into your vagina to lubricate and promote the absorption of water into vaginal tissues; castor oil and olive oil also work well if applied daily and prior to intercourse. Replens, if applied regularly, will make your vagina more supple. A randomized controlled study comparing Replens with vaginal estrogen found that both were equally effective in treating vaginal dryness.

Exploring Your Fantasies Share your fantasies with your partner or keep them to yourself to enhance your desire or mood. Try creating a fantasy with your partner.

Learning Your Pleasure Points There are many ways to learn your erogenous zones. Self-stimulation or self-massage is a good way to learn about your pleasure points. Try mutual masturbation as part of your foreplay to help you both learn what kind of touch turns each other on. Buy a vibrator and experiment with it on yourself when you're alone and with your partner as part of foreplay.

Using Aphrodisiac Scents In one study, women considered smell the most important factor in selecting a mate. For women, aphrodisiac scents are rose maroc, ylang-ylang, jasmine, sandalwood, patchouli, benzoin, and pimento. These scents are considered aphrodisiacs because they stimulate the human pheromones, or sexual attractants men emit from glands in their armpits and groin. You can find essential oils at your local health food or herb store. Try this blend and see if it puts you in the mood: three drops rose maroc, three drops nutmeg, two drops bergamot, four drops vanilla. Blend with a half-ounce of vegetable or almond oil. Use as a body lotion or put three drops in your bath and invite your partner to join you.

Having Regular Sex Having regular sex can keep your vagina from shrinking. If you don't have a partner or if your vagina has already shrunk, purchase a vibrator and use your finger to slowly expand and stimulate your vagina.

Trying New Sexual Positions There's no right way to have intercourse. Buy a book that describes different positions and experiment. Find one or more you're both comfortable with and add it to your repertoire.

Making a Date for Love Setting aside a date for lovemaking may not be spontaneous, but it gives you an opportunity to have fun planning. What will you wear? What scent will you use? How will you fix your hair? To increase your anticipation, abstain from intercourse for at least several days before you rendezvous.

Creating a Romantic Interlude Increase the drama of your lovemaking by planning a special Sunday morning with French toast or strawberry muffins—in bed. On a rainy day, crawl in bed and watch a sexy movie as a prelude to lovemaking. Put on your favorite music, fresh flowers on the night table, and massage each other's feet with a scented oil.

Getting Some Instruction You can never learn too much. Rent a movie or check out a book that is evocative. Browse the shelves of your local bookstore or library for a new sex manual. Call the Sinclair Institute at (800) 955-0888 to obtain a catalog of videos, including *The Better Sex Video Series* and *The Couples' Guide to Great Sex Over 40*. You can also contact the Virginia Johnson Masters Learning Center at (888) 937-3528 or visit the Learning Center at http://www.vjmlc.com.

Using Homeopathic Remedies Graphites is one homeopathic remedy used by those with an aversion to sex. It can be used in a 12C or 30C dilution daily until improvement occurs.

■ Skin Problems

Avoid:

Triggering Cosmetics Cosmetics can cause scaling and swelling characteristic of dermatitis. Dermatologist Susan T. Nedorost of Cleveland's Case Western Reserve University said in a presentation to the American Academy of Dermatology that tracking down just which one is triggering reactions can be difficult because the reaction may not show up for several days after contact. Fragrances and preservatives in toiletries are the most common triggers. Triggers also include chemicals in makeup pads and foam applicators, eyelash curlers, tweezers and earrings, artificial nails, mascara, shampoo, and sunscreens. Your best course is to stop using cosmetics containing triggering chemicals. Keep a skin/cosmetic diary. Wear nothing for several days then add cosmetics back one by one until you identify the offending product(s).

Focus On:

Oatmeal Oatmeal extract can decrease swelling and dilated vessels in the skin. Find a body lotion that contains oatmeal extract and try it.

Other Topicals Chamomile can be used to soothe skin, promote new growth, and bring relief. Other healing herbs that can be added to castor or almond oil to make a healing body lotion include comfrey, aloe vera gel, calendula, chickweed, and arnica.

Pine Tar Soap Pine tar has been used for skin conditions of many kinds. Find a bar at your local health food store and try it.

Drinking Water Staying well hydrated is key to healthy skin. If you carry around a plastic water bottle, make sure it doesn't have a 1 inside the recycling symbol on the bottom. If it does, it's only meant for one-time use. After that, the plastic may start to break down and leach into the water. Summer heat is apt to speed up this process. Even if you wash your bottles frequently, you may not be able to prevent bacteria from building up. Find a hard plastic bottle, or better yet, bring a tall glass to work to keep on your desk instead of a water bottle.

■ Urinary Symptoms

Avoid:

Aluminum Cookware   Using aluminum cookware may cause cystitis.

Contaminating Your Bladder   Never wipe from back to front. Always wipe from front to back so that you don't transfer bacteria to your bladder.

Toxic Metals   Cadmium and other toxic metals can cause urinary problems. Drink only distilled water or water that has been processed through a reverse osmosis filter.

Focus On:

Good Bladder Hygiene   Empty your bladder every 2 to 3 waking hours. Set a timer if necessary. Sit in the bathtub in warm water that covers your hips for 20 minutes twice a day. Add 1 cup of vinegar to the water. Position your knees up and apart so the water can enter the vagina. Alternate this with a bath made with two cloves of crushed garlic. Use only a mild, nondeodorant and fragrance-free soap or just plain water.

Soothing Baths   Soaking in a soothing baking soda or oatmeal bath can be an effective treatment for painful urination due to urinary tract, bladder, or vaginal infection or irritation. Add 1 cup of baking soda or oatmeal to a warm water bath and soak for 15 minutes.

Staying Dry   Thoroughly dry yourself after a shower or bath; dampness can cause bacteria to multiply. Wear panties made of cotton, which "breathes" and lets moisture evaporate.

Yogurt Douche Rub a teaspoon worth of plain yogurt around the outside of your vagina, urethra, and labia. This will help neutralize acidic body fluids that can lead to painful urination.

■ Weight Gain

Avoid:

Weight Gain Situations Impulse buying or shopping on an empty stomach, alcohol, skipping meals, crash dieting, and using large serving plates.

Focus On:

Reorganizing Your Kitchen Toss out foods that contain trans-fats such as hydrogenated or partially hydrogenated vegetable oil or shortening (you'll find them in most crackers, cookies, and packaged foods; they are associated with hardening of the arteries, some types of cancer, eczema, arthritis, irritable bowel syndrome, and more), high-sugar foods, highly processed foods including white flour products, and food containing additives such as artificial colors and flavors and preservatives. Stock your shelves with soy, organically grown fruits and vegetables, and whole-grain cereals and breads.

Exercise

Exercise is the closest thing to a miracle treatment. It can help you maintain a youthful and healthy body, help you ward off chronic conditions, energize you, and reduce anxiety and depression. This chapter presents some of the ways you can use exercise to make your menopause experience the most positive it can be.

There are several types of exercise. *Range-of-motion exercise,* such as circling your arms, helps you maintain shoulder joint movement. *Strengthening and toning exercise* strengthens and tones a specific muscle or set of muscles, such as sit-ups for your abdominal muscles, weight training that tightens many parts of the body, or contracting specific pelvis muscles to strengthen control of your bladder, bowels, and vagina. *Aerobic or endurance exercise* includes rhythmic, sustained movement, like walking or cycling, and can benefit your heart and blood vessels, lower blood pressure, and lift mood.

A total exercise program includes warming up the body, then completing aerobic and strengthening or toning exercises. It's important to select activities that you look forward to doing, whether you use an exercise video, attend a class, or exercise with a buddy. Whatever you choose, start out slowly, listen to your body, and gradually increase the duration and intensity of your workout. You should not feel pain or stiffness or struggle to breathe. If you do, you're overexercising, and you may need to join a class, hire a trainer, or use an exercise video that suits you. If you've been sedentary for some time, consult with your health care provider before beginning an exercise program.

> *Jennifer, age 49, had been postmenopausal for 7 years when I first met her. She worked part-time as a legal assistant. She said her hot flashes were more consistent taking Premarin (mare's urine), but it didn't help her back pain or the arthritis in her fingers. She'd tried Tylenol but was worried that she might be getting addicted to the drug. She tried to exercise but didn't do so more than once every week or two. We devised a plan for her to partner with another client to walk every morning before work. She lost 10 of the 30 pounds she'd gained within the first month and reported sleeping better and having fewer hot flashes. She also told me she thought exercising helped make her less "emotional."*

Below you'll find some exercise recommendations that could help you.

■ Breast Cancer and Other Cancers

Avoid:
Inactivity   Cancer is more prevalent among inactive people.

Focus On:
The Female Deer Exercise   This exercise has been used for thousands of years by Taoist practitioners to prevent or cure lumps and cancer of the breasts.

1. Sit down in a quiet, relaxing spot.
2. Rub your hands together vigorously. This will create heat and bring the energy of your body into your palms.
3. Place your hands on your breasts.
4. Rub clockwise with your right hand and counterclockwise with your left hand, finishing at your side. Avoid touching the nipples as they are very sensitive. Repeat for a minimum of 36 times and a maximum of 360 times once or twice a day. This inward circular rubbing is called *dispersion*.

Walking Away from Breast Cancer   If you exercise, you're much less likely to develop breast cancer and other cancers. At least 45 minutes of moderate to vigorous exercise five times a week may be required. This can help burn up the stored fat that produces estrogen, which in turn can fuel breast cancer growth.

Even a little bit of exercise can help. In one study, women who walked 3 mph lowered their risk of dying from breast cancer by one-quarter, compared to the most sedentary women. Those who walked between three and eight hours a week cut their risk in half.

In another study conducted by the Fred Hutchinson Cancer Research Center in Seattle, Washington, women who engaged in 1.25 to 2.5 hours per week of brisk walking had an 18% decreased risk of breast cancer compared with inactive women. Slightly greater reduction in risk was observed for women who exercised 10 hours or more per week by walking briskly. The good news is that the activity need not be strenuous to provide protection.

■ Cold Hands

Avoid:

Inactivity   Not moving decreases vital circulation to the extremities.

Focus On:

Finger Pulls Finger pulls—a yoga exercise—bring circulation and strength to your fingers, shoulders, back, chest, upper arms, and forearms.

1. Either sit on a chair or on the floor, keeping your back straight and head erect. Breathe slowly and deeply through your nose while doing the yoga movements in these steps.
2. Bend your elbows and bring your hands in level with your chest. Turn the palm of the left hand away from you and grip your thumb firmly with your right hand.
3. Pull both hands in toward you and down, moving slowly and firmly, releasing the thumb at the level of your navel.
4. Repeat the movement with the other fingers of the left hand and then change hands.

■ Depression, Nervousness, and Irritability

Avoid:

Inactivity During inactivity the brain doesn't produce feel-good chemicals called endorphins and enkephalins that produce a natural "high."

Focus On:

Walking In one study, a 6-minute walk reduced depressive symptoms. In another study, older adults showed a reduction in depression after an exercise training program.

Yoga Yogis believe that if you expose your armpits several times a day, you will not get depressed. The Triangle is an exercise you can do to expose your armpits. The movement also brings nourishing blood to your brain and face, elongating the sides of your body, firming the torso as well as the legs and arms. The Triangle also gives you an incredible feeling of power and strength.

1. Stand with feet approximately 2 feet apart and raise your arms to shoulder level.
2. Breathe through the nose, bringing in refreshing and calming energy.
3. Keeping your elbows and knees straight straight, slowly slide your right arm down your right leg as far as you can easily reach. (Your eventual target is to place your fingertips on the floor, but the knee or shin is fine for now.)
4. Bring your left arm over your ear and look up at the palm, stretching your head and neck up while stretching down with the right hand.
5. Hold for at least a count of 5.
6. Straighten up and repeat on the other side.

■ Dizziness

Avoid:
Rapid or Extreme Movements Rapid changes in body position and extreme movements can bring on dizziness.

Focus On:
Cawthorne-Cooksey Exercises

Rachel, age 50, hadn't had a period for two years, and her health care provider proclaimed her postmenopausal. Rachel's hot flashes were under control, but she began to suffer from dizziness, for which her provider could find no physical cause. I told Rachel about the Cawthorne-Cooksey exercises and she tried them. They reduced her dizziness and increased her balance.

Research has demonstrated that the Cawthorne-Cooksey Exercises can decrease dizziness and enhance balance. Try them.

1. Sitting in bed or in a chair, use your eyes only to look slowly to the left and the right, then quickly up and down and from side to side, focusing on one of your fingers moving from 3 feet to 1 foot away from your face.
2. Move your head, first slowly, then quickly, later with eyes closed, bending forward and backward, turning from side to side.
3. Shrug your shoulders while circling them, bending forward and picking up objects from the ground.
4. Standing, repeat steps 2 and 3 with eyes open, then shut.
5. Throw a small ball from hand to hand and then under your knee, changing from sitting to standing and turning around in between.
6. Move around a person who plays catch with you, using a large ball.
7. Walk across the room with eyes open and then closed.
8. Walk up and down a slope with eyes open and then closed.
9. Walk up and down steps with eyes open and then closed.
10. Play any game involving stooping, stretching, and aiming, such as bowling or basketball.

Diligence and perseverance are required, but the earlier and more regularly the exercise regimen is carried out, the faster and more complete will be the return to normal activity. Ideally these activities should be done with a supervised group. Individual exercises should only be tried in the presence of a vigilant friend or relative who also learns the exercises and can help you.

■ Fatigue

Avoid:

Inactivity   A sedentary lifestyle can lead to poor muscle tone, decreased metabolism, and fatigue.

Focus On:

Aerobic Exercise At least one study showed that aerobic exercise has a positive effect on fatigue. Whether you choose walking, cycling, dancing, or some other rhythmic and sustained effort, exercising can energize you and reduce fatigue.

Shiatsu Shiatsu includes using the fingers to create pressure and enhance circulation. To relieve fatigue, press the bottom of each foot in the middle for 1 minute using a spiral movement.

■ Hair Loss/Thinning

Avoid:

Inactivity Inactivity can lead to poor circulation, which is correlated with hair loss.

Focus On:

Massage Massage can increase circulation to your scalp and improve hair quality. Massage your scalp at least once a day, covering every inch of your head. Use your fingertips to make small circles. If your hair is dry, use jojoba or olive oil. Also grab a handful of hair and gently tug, keeping your fingers tight, against your scalp to increase circulation and strengthen scalp.

High-Touch Energy Release Points High Touch is a self-healing art born in ancient oriental traditions. This method uses a kind of gentle acupressure that finds and holds pulsations throughout the body to open energy channels so natural healing can occur. Find a quiet spot and sit or lie down in a comfortable place.

1. Hold the little finger of one hand with your index, third, and fourth fingers just tight enough so you can feel a pulsation in each of the three fingers. Hold until ready to release. Repeat with the little finger of the other hand.

2. Hold the thumb of one hand as in step 1. Repeat with the other hand.
3. Hold the index finger of one hand as in step 1. Repeat with the other hand.

■ Headaches

Avoid:

Inactivity   Tension and poor circulation are increased by inactivity.

Focus On:

Acupressure   Use the tips of your fingers to press on the points below. Use enough pressure to make the point hurt a bit. Press the points for 15 to 30 seconds, decreasing the pressure every few seconds but not removing your fingers.

Point 1: Work at the middle base of your skull with your thumbs side by side.

Point 2: Find a small hollow on the outer edge of each eye socket. Press with your index fingers.

(The next two points are especially for sinus and tension headaches.)

Point 3: Press the point where the nose bridge meets the brow. Use your thumb and index finger to press the point, then hold and breathe deeply for a minute or two.

Point 4: Squeeze the webbing between the thumb and index finger. Breathe deeply while pressing for 1 minute. Repeat on the other hand. Do not use this point if you are in the early stages of pregnancy; some experts believe it could have a negative effect.

Gently pound the top of the head with your fist many times. Also pound at the hairline. This causes contraction and is effective for expansive headaches. Lightly pound the shoulders down the neck to the arms and back again, then press with the thumbs across the top of the shoulders. Repeat as long as it feels good.

Aerobic Exercise One study evaluated the effect of exercise on migraines. Forty participants with headaches exercised on a treadmill and were asked to continue an aerobic home exercise program for 6 weeks. Exercise was found to have beneficial effects on all migraine parameters, increasing endorphin levels after treadmill practice and after the home exercise. Exercise does not only provide ongoing protection for migraines but protection for other headaches as well because of the neurochemicals that are released.

Isometric Neck Exercise The New York Headache Center in New York recommends isometric neck exercise for headaches. These exercises are more effective when performed in the shower or after the application of hot moist towels. They help restore motion and relieve pain associated with stiffness.

1. Stand erect. Turn your head slowly to the right as far as possible without straining. Return to normal center position. Repeat on the other side.
2. Try to touch your right ear to your right shoulder. Return to normal center position. Repeat with your left ear and left shoulder.
3. Raise both shoulders as close to the ears as possible and hold for a count of 5. Relax. Stretch your shoulders backward as far as possible and hold, then relax.
4. Try to touch your chin to your chest. Rotate your head backward slowly, looking up at the ceiling.

■ Heart Disease

Avoid:

Inactivity Sedentary people are at high risk for heart attack.

Focus On:

Arm Massage   These exercises are like those practiced in tai chi, kung fu, and karate. They build up strength in the arms and hands, tone muscles and nerves, increase blood circulation, and energize the heart, lung, and heart meridians along the arm.

1. Sit or stand and place the left palm on the inside of your right shoulder.
2. Using a continuous movement, rub your palm down the inside of your arm, elbow, and out the tips of your fingers.
3. Rub up the back of your right hand and elbow until you reach your shoulder.
4. Repeat 12 times.
5. Follow steps 1 through 4 with the left arm.

Leg Rubbing   According to Dr. Stephen T. Chang, this exercise works the upward meridians of the legs, helping to dispel the energy from the body, which is why it helps with problems such as water retention and high blood pressure. It is best done in the morning to energize your body.

1. Stand, sit, or lie down. Breathe naturally through the entire exercise.
2. Place the palms of your hands on the inside of your ankles.
3. In a continuous movement, rub your hands up the inside of your legs from your ankles to the top of your thighs.
4. Repeat 12 times.

Walking   In one study, 20 postmenopausal women at risk for coronary artery disease were placed on a high-fiber, low-fat diet and daily aerobic exercise, primarily walking. Overall, the program resulted in improved metabolic and blood fats and reduced inflammation. The researchers concluded these improvements may reduce the risk of acute heart attack (myocardial infarction). If sustained, these changes could reduce the risk for atherosclerosis (hardening of the arteries).

Researchers in another study put 114 overweight older women on an exercise program and monitored their levels of C-reactive protein (CRP). High CRP levels are a sign of inflammation and an indicator of heart disease. After a year of brisk walking, CRP levels fell even in the women who didn't lose much weight.

■ Hot Flashes

Avoid:
Inactivity

Focus On:
Exercising   Physically active women have 50% fewer hot flashes than women who are sedentary. It should be noted that until you become conditioned and your body adjusts, strenuous exercise that causes perspiration may trigger hot flashes. Work through this stage if you want results, but use slow walking and other forms of gentle exercise that don't make you sweat.

■ Insomnia/Sleep Problems

Focus On:
Exercising in the Morning   A study conducted at the Fred Hutchinson Cancer Research Center in Seattle, Washington, examined the effects of a moderate-intensity exercise or stretching program on fitness, body mass index, or time spent outdoors on self-reported sleep quality. Postmenopausal overweight sedentary women aged 50 to 75 participated in a year-long moderate-intensity exercise and low-intensity stretching program. Among morning ex-

ercisers, those who exercised at least 225 minutes (3.75 hours) a week had less trouble falling asleep compared with those who exercised less than 180 minutes (3 hours) a week. Among evening exercisers, women who exercised at least 225 minutes a week had more trouble falling asleep compared with those who exercised less than 180 minutes a week. The researchers concluded that both stretching and exercise can improve sleep quality, and increased fitness was associated with improvements in sleep, but the effects may depend on the amount of exercise and time of day it is performed. Exercising in the morning is better if you want to sleep.

■ Itchiness

Avoid:
Tight, Nonporous Exercise Clothes   Restrictive clothes can bring on itchiness.

Focus On:
Wearing Loose, Porous Exercise Clothing
Movement   Just moving around can help if itchiness is due to poor circulation.

■ Joint and Muscle Pain

Avoid:
Straining or Overdoing

Focus On:
Massage and Walking   Rubbing the legs or walking have been determined to bring relief from restless leg syndrome.
6-Minute Walk   The Arthritis, Diet and Activity Promotion Trial (ADAPT) study lasted 18 months and was designed to determine

whether long-term exercise (6 minutes of walking daily) and dietary weight loss are more effective, either separately or in combination, than usual care in improving physical function, pain, and mobility in older overweight adults with knee osteoarthritis. Three hundred sixteen community-dwelling adults 60 years and older who had knee pain were randomly assigned to diet only, exercise only, diet plus exercise, or healthy lifestyle (a control group that received neither additional diet nor exercise assistance). Only the exercise group and diet plus exercise group showed significant improvements in self-reported physical function and knee pain.

Pain Busters Strong muscles act as shock absorbers that help protect your joints. When you have weak muscles, your joints aren't that stable and pain can result. Try one or more of the exercises that follow:

1. *Strengthen thighs and buttocks:* Stand with your feet hip-width apart, toes our slightly, arms crossed. Bend your knees and lower yourself to a chair, then push up. Work up to 12 repetitions.

2. *Strengthen shoulders and upper body:* Lie on the floor on a mat or carpet with a 2.5 or 10-pound weight in each hand held shoulder high. Keep elbows slightly bent and hips and back flat on the floor. Bring arms up until weights almost touch, then return. Work up to two sets of 12 repetitions with a 30-second rest between sets. If you're out of shape, practice without weights. As you get stronger, gradually increase the weights.

3. *Strengthen back by strengthening abs:* Your abdominal muscles support your back. If they're weak, you're apt to have backaches. Sit on a mat or carpet, legs bent, hands on the floor, fingers facing forward, feet flat on the floor. Raise your hands and grab your legs below your knees. Hold for 3–5 seconds, increasing the time as you grow stronger.

4. *Strengthen knees:* Sit in a chair, knees bent, then straighten one leg and raise it. Pause when it's parallel to the floor and return to starting position. Work up to 12 repetitions, rest 30 seconds, and do another set of 12. As you get stronger, add 1- to 3-pound ankle weights. You can also stand with feet and knees together. Bend your knees enough so you can easily circle knees and ankles, working up to 10 circles.

5. *Strengthen hips:* Stand and circle hips, exaggerating the movement. Work up to 10 circles in each direction.

■ Memory Loss and Foggy Thinking

Avoid:
Being Sedentary

Focus On:
Walking In one study, memory increased after participants walked for 6 minutes compared with a control group that didn't walk.

■ Menstrual Bleeding

Avoid:
Inactivity Lying around or sitting in front of the TV is not a good idea during a menstrual period. Walking, even half a mile a day, can help stabilize hormones, and increase oxygen level in the blood, which helps in nutrient absorption, and elimination of toxins.

Focus On:
Gentle Exercise According to Dr. M. R. Richardson of the University of Kansas Medical Center, gentle exercise combined with weight loss can help control irregular bleeding. Gentle exercise

could include slow walking, slow dancing, easy gardening, or slow biking on a flat road.

Acupressure   Consider acupressure to control bleeding.

1. Using the palms of your hands press 1½ inches on each side of the spine moving up to the shoulders. Hold for 2–5 seconds at each point.

2. Place one hand, palm down, on the navel and the other hand directly on top. Breathe in a deep, full breath, and on exhalation press gently down until you find resistance. Hold for 1–5 seconds. Repeat at least 10 times. Finish by massaging the entire area with the heel of your hand.

3. Massage the bottom of your feet and then around the ankles and just below the knees on the inside. Any tender spots are worth massaging a little more.

■ Osteoporosis

Avoid:

Participating in Non-Weight-Bearing Exercise   Swimming is an example of the kind of exercise that does not build bone mass and cannot protect against osteoporosis.

Yoga   There are several yoga movements that can help strengthen bones and stretch the back, keeping it limber.

1. Lie flat on your back with legs and feet together and arms by your side. Moving very slowly, reach forward with your arms. Bring your hands down to your legs and let your chin drop to your chest. Start to roll slowly back down, keeping your elbows straight, hands pointing toward your toes, and shoulders hunched. After your back touches the floor, let your head go back and lie flat for a few seconds. Repeat the whole movement four times. Repeat twice daily.

2. Lie on your back with legs and feet together and palms flat on the floor. Bend your knees, interlock your fingers, and pull your knees toward your chest. Raise your head toward your knees. Hold for a count of 5. Lower your head and relax, still holding your knees. Repeat twice, then undo your fingers and lie flat on the floor again.

3. Inhale deeply while raising your arms until your hands meet straight above your head. Exhale, lowering your arms slowly back to your sides. Let your hands brush the floor as you raise and lower them. Repeat the entire movement eight times.

4. Get on the floor on your hands and knees. Slowly arch your back like a cat, then let your back sink down, raising your head. Continue to arch the back and bow it five times. When finished, sit back on your heels and remain with your head bowed for a few moments. Then repeat the cat twice more.

5. Go to the Joint and Muscle Pain section and complete step 3 under Pain Busters.

Weight-Bearing Exercise Tai chi, weightlifting, and bike riding are examples of weight-bearing exercises that build bone and strengthen muscle.

■ Sex Drive Reduction or Intercourse Discomfort

Avoid:
Muscle Weakness in Your Pelvis

Focus On:
Abdominal Contractions This exercise will tighten up the pelvic floor, toning your uterus and vagina. Without exercise, these muscles can become slack. Lie in bed on your back with legs, feet, arms, and hands completely relaxed. Pull your abdomen in and up as much as possible and hold for a slow count of 5. Relax the muscles

and wait a few seconds before repeating. Perform the contraction movement six times, twice a day. With practice, gradually increase holding for a slow count of 10.

Kegels   Although Kegels are best known for controlling urine flow, the muscle that is exercised during that movement is the same one that contracts during orgasm. Like any muscle, unless it is exercised, its function is reduced with age. To enhance circulation and your sexual experiences, imagine you're urinating (or actually urinate) and stop the flow midstream. Notice which muscle you use to do this. Tighten this muscle again, hold for 10 seconds, then release. Repeat up to 10 times or more daily. Contract this muscle during intercourse to bring more pleasure to your partner.

Shiatsu   To help your partner (or yourself) bring a strong blood supply to the genital area, press lightly along the base of the spine from the tailbone up to waist level. At each point, press for 3 seconds and give 10 applications. Also press three fingers into a point located directly on the midline of the abdomen an inch or two under the breastbone. This is believed to promote sexual energy. Try the top border of the public hair using gentle pressure. Ask your partner to apply firm but gentle palm pressure to the area where your leg joins the hip, then to press along the sacrum between the buttocks. To learn more about these methods, find a Shiatsu practitioner or a Shiatsu wall chart that shows pressure points.

■ Skin Problems

Avoid:
Being Sedentary   Lack of movement decreases circulation and reduces nourishment to skin cells.

Focus On:
Front Push-Ups   This exercise improves the complexion by allowing blood to flow freely into your face. Hold the positions for a

count of 5. You may shake a little during the count. If you do, reduce to a count of 3 until your arms strengthen.

1. Get on your hands and knees. Tuck your toes under so that you are resting on the balls of the feet. Bend your elbows so your nose comes down toward the floor.
2. Take a deep breath in through your nose and push up, straightening the elbows and the knees, allowing your head to relax completely, letting it hang. While you move, continue to breathe slowly and normally.
3. Slowly lower your knees and return to starting position, keeping your head relaxed.
4. Repeat.
5. Relax with knees bent beneath you, arms along your sides, and forehead on the floor (fetal position).

Standing Leg Grip The following exercise stretches the back and neck and allows fresh blood to flow into your head and face, bringing healing circulation.

1. Stand with the legs and feet about 2 feet apart and let your arms, hands, and head hang completely limp.
2. Grip your legs at the point where your arms hang relaxed, and raise your head slightly, keeping your elbows straight.
3. While taking a deep breath through your nose, pull on the legs, letting your elbows go out to the side, and bring your head in as far as you can. Hold the position for a count of 5.
4. Straighten your elbows slowly, exhale, and raise your head up a few inches. Breathe normally for a few seconds while you relax. Repeat. When you finish, let your head and arms hang completely limp, then slowly straighten up, bringing your head up last.

Elevating Your Feet Lie on the floor and put your feet on a bench or a triangular pillow that elevates your feet and legs above the level of your heart. Lie relaxed for 15–20 minutes twice daily. This will bring blood to your chest and face.

Weight Training According to David Pearson, director of the Strength Research Laboratory at Ball State University, pushing and pulling weights tightens many parts of the body, particularly face and neck muscles. This keeps the skin from looking loose and droopy. Consider joining a gym that offers weight training supervision or buy a book on weight training such as Joyce Vedral's *Definition: Shape Without Bulk in 15 Minutes a Day!*

Removing and Preventing Facial Wrinkles Facial wrinkles develop most readily in areas where the muscle beneath is thin and movements of the face are small and frequent, including the forehead, the ends of the eyes, and the neck. Do the next four exercises every time you wash, apply cleanser, moisturize, or apply makeup. Try for at least twice a day.

Form a large O with your mouth and close your eyes. Hold this position throughout all the steps, breathing in and out through your nose in a calm fashion.

1. Trace a circle around the eyes using the fingertips of both hands and moving from the inner corners of your eyes, up and around. Complete 10 times, working up to 50–60 times.
2. Massage your nose in a downward fashion five times.
3. Massage in a full circle around your mouth five times, then five times in the opposite direction.
4. Using 5 to 10 long strokes, massage from the bridge of the nose upward and outward over your forehead to your hairline.

Firming the Lower Part of Your Face Stand in front of a mirror.

1. Roll your lips inward over your upper and lower teeth. Keep your mouth open about half an inch. Smile as widely as you can with your lower jaw. Keep the rest of your face still.

2. Massage the entire lower part of your face using a small outward circling movement. Start at the tip of the chin, moving up to your ears and back down again to a slow count of 10–20.

Rejuvenating Your Neck

1. Place your thumb under the middle of your chin and hold.
2. Curl your tongue back in your mouth until you find the spot where your thumb is on the outside.
3. Release your thumb, but keep your tongue curled.
4. Tilt your head back and stretch your neck as far as possible to the left to a slow count of 10.
5. Repeat, tilting your head to the right.
6. Place all fingertips at the base of your neck and massage in vigorous, long, upward strokes up to your jawbone to a slow count of 10 while moving your head in a half-circle arc from left to right.

Firming Mouth and Filling Out Lips Make a small O with your mouth. Pucker harder and harder. Slowly massage in tiny outward circles around your mouth.

■ Urinary Symptoms

Avoid:

Retaining the Urine in the Bladder for Long Periods Going to the toilet to empty the bladder can protect against bladder infections and possibly bladder cancer.

Focus On:

Kegels Lie on your back, stand up, or sit. Contract the vagina and feel the same sort of sensation as when you stop your urine flow. Hold for a few seconds, relax, and repeat up to 100 times a day.

■ Weight Gain

Avoid:
A Sedentary Lifestyle

Focus On:
Leg Rubbing Sit in a chair stand or lie down and lean forward. In a continuous movement, rub your hands down the outside of your legs from the top of your thighs to your ankles. Repeat 12 times. This exercise helps dispel energy from the body by activating the gallbladder, bladder, and stomach meridians, which is why it helps treat overweight, water retention, and high blood pressure.

Abdominal Contractions

1. Sit or lie in bed with legs, feet, arms, and hands completely relaxed.
2. Pull your abdomen in and up as far as you can and hold for a slow count of 5.
3. Relax for a few seconds and repeat up to six times twice a day, gradually increasing the holding count to 10.

Alternate Leg Raise This exercise firms and tones the legs, thighs, and tummy.

1. Sit in bed, resting your back against a couple of firm pillows.
2. Keeping your knee straight, and raise your right leg a few inches. Hold for a count of 5.
3. Lower the leg slowly, keeping your knee straight.

4. Repeat with your left leg.
5. Repeat twice more with each leg twice a day, working up to holding for a count of 10.

Standing Slide Bend This gentle exercise will reduce excess weight from the waist and streamline your torso. It can also eliminate stiffness from the neck and improve balance.

1. Stand straight with legs and feet together, palms flat against your legs, and head erect. Inhale through your nose.
2. Holding your breath, slowly bend right, sliding your right hand down toward the knee, letting your left hand slide up toward the hip, head relaxing to the right and hanging down limp for a count of 5 while you exhale.
3. Relax your head forward; inhale and exhale through the nose.
4. Repeat step 2 only on the left side.

Rub Your Stomach Away: The Crane The final exercise will help melt away menopause belly. By bringing circulation to the area and stimulating peristalsis, digestion and elimination are improved. The exercise is also soothing and calming, reducing the stress that often fuels binge-eating and overweight.

1. Lie flat on your back.
2. Put your writing hand on your navel.
3. Rub clockwise from the center in small, gradually expanding circles until the upper and lower limits of your abdomen are being rubbed. Use slow, gentle pressure.
4. Reverse the movement, rubbing in smaller and smaller counterclockwise circles until you reach the navel.

8

Other Stress Reduction and Healing Measures

Bridget, 52 years old and in the throes of menopause, faced the stresses of running a nursing department, raising her granddaughter, and taking care of her mom who was recently diagnosed with Alzheimer's disease. Bridget came to see me because she felt "stressed out." I taught her relaxation, self-hypnosis, and guided-imagery procedures. A month later, she reported feeling "much calmer." She was also surprised how much the procedures reduced her hot flashes and helped with her muscle pain and urge to urinate. She even started to sleep through the night, which she hadn't been able to do since before her daughter was born.

There are many stress reduction and healing measures that can help you. Some of the better-known and researched ones are presented below.

■ Breast Cancer and Other Cancers

Avoid:
Non-Supportive People and Distressing Touch

Focus On:
Stress Reduction, Comforting Touch, and Good Listeners Stress can influence cancer. A study of women with breast cancer published in the *Journal of the National Cancer Institute* found that women who were taught stress reduction techniques achieved a greater reduction in hot flashes, vaginal dryness, and stress incontinence than their counterparts with breast cancer who received no instruction. Other researchers found that women who were listened to by a concerned, empathetic nurse, or who received therapeutic touch, expressed feelings of calmness, relaxation, security, and comfort.

Hypnotic Guided Imagery Studies have shown that hypnotic guided imagery can have a positive effect on psychological well-being and immune function. To use hypnotic guided imagery, complete steps 5 and 6 for hypnosis. When you feel relaxed, keep your eyes closed and picture your breasts functioning perfectly. Give yourself the suggestion that your breasts are getting healthier and healthier. Repeat this procedure until you are able to picture your breasts healthy inside and out. The changes may not be retained after your self-treatment ends, so continue to use hypnotic guided imagery to maintain positive effects.

■ Cold Hands

Avoid:
Shallow Breathing Cold hands and feet are common symptoms of stress. When you're stressed you breathe in your upper chest, and your arteries constrict, carrying blood away from your core. The

more stressed you are, the colder your hands. The objective of stress reduction techniques is to reduce stressful thoughts and bring circulation back to your hands.

Focus On:

Positive Imagery Find a quiet room and sit in a chair or lie on the floor with your palms facing upward. Take slow-paced breaths for a minute or two. Picture yourself relaxing. Feel your feet getting heavy and relaxed. Feel your knees getting heavy and relaxed. Feel your hips getting heavy and relaxed. Feel the center of your body relaxing. Let all your internal organs spread out and relax, taking up all the space available to them. Feel your shoulders relaxing. Picture a relaxing color running across your shoulders, down your arms, and out your fingertips warming your hands. Picture your neck relaxing, your head and brain relaxing, your scalp and hair relaxing, your eyes and nose relaxing. Scan your body, find areas that need more relaxing, and send a wave of relaxation to those areas the next time you exhale.

Hypnosis Studies have shown that hypnosis, using suggestions to increase the warmth in your hands, can increase fingertip skin temperature. Hypnosis works the best when warmth suggestions include experiences of physical temperature and relaxation—for example, saying or hearing, "Your hands are feeling warm and relaxed."

■ Depression, Nervousness, and Irritability

Avoid:
Negative Thinking

Focus On:
Bibliotherapy (Reading Books) A total of 31 adults received either 16 sessions of individual cognitive psychotherapy or read *Feel-*

ing Good, The New Mood Therapy by Dr. David Burns. Individual psychotherapy was superior to bibliotherapy on self-reported depression, but there were no differences in clinician-rated depression. Bibliotherapy participants continued to improve after treatment, and at 3-month follow-up there were no differences between treatments. The findings suggest that bibliotherapy and individual psychotherapy are both viable treatment options for depression.

Cognitive-Behavioral Techniques Your anxious or depressed mood is probably associated with negative thinking. In fact, negative thinking has been shown to precede negative feelings. For this reason, it's important to identify negative thinking patterns. Cognitive-behavioral approaches emphasize the identification and modification of distorted thinking patterns. *Self-talk* describes the ongoing internal conversations you have with yourself every waking moment. Over the years you probably developed some negative self-talk. Your mood will improve when your self-talk becomes more positive.

Check which of the following styles applies to your self-talk:

❏ 1. *Filtering or "awfulizing."* You focus on a negative aspect of a situation and allow this detail to color your feelings. You use words such as *awful, terrible,* and *horrible.*

❏ 2. *Overgeneralization.* You reach a conclusion based on a single incident or piece of evidence and use words such as *always, never, nobody,* and *everyone.*

❏ 3. *Black-or-white thinking.* You see everything as an extreme and anything short of perfection is failure.

❏ 4. *Labeling.* You focus on only one aspect or quality in yourself, a situation, or other people, calling yourself or others names such as *stupid* and *jerk.*

❏ 5. *Mind reading.* You make negative assumptions about other people and their actions with little or no evidence to support your conclusions—for example, assuming a look from someone else means you're boring or dumb.

❑ 6. *Catastrophizing.* You make negative assumptions about the future—for example, a headache becomes a sign of a brain tumor and a sore breast a symptom of cancer.

❑ 7. *Personalizing.* You relate everything that occurs around you to yourself, comparing yourself to others or blaming yourself for an outcome that you didn't have anything to do with.

❑ 8. *Using "shoulds."* You tell yourself what you should have done or what you must do. The emotional consequence is feeling guilty no matter what you do. When you direct should statements toward others, you feel anger, frustration, and resentment because they don't live up to your expectations.

❑ 9. *Emotional reasoning.* You believe that your negative emotions really reflect how things are, telling yourself, "I feel bad, so this must be how things are."

Now that you have a handle on the distorted patterns that probably feed your negative moods, what can be done? Here are some ideas:

- Train yourself to challenge the self-critical comments you make.
- Identify self-critical or automatic thoughts you have about being wrong, stupid, a jerk, feeling you'll be looked down on by others, or not being perfect.
- Purchase a diary and divide each page into three columns. Write your self-critical or automatic thoughts in the left column—for example, "This is horrible. I should be able to get places on time. I'm always late. Can't I ever do anything right? Everyone will know about me now and see what a jerk I am." Identify which cognitive distortions you're using (see the list above) in the middle column. In this case, awfulizing, shoulds, overgeneralization, and labeling are used.

- Write down more rational responses to your self-critical comments in the right column—for example, "I'm not always late. That's ridiculous. I was late last week and a month ago, but that's it. Everyone's late once in a while. I'm going to make a plan so that I won't be late again and follow it; that will take care of the problem."

Writing   Writing can be a powerful way to reduce anxiety, depression, and irritability. Although writing about an upsetting event has been shown in numerous studies to reduce negative feelings, you can write about mundane things (such as what you're having for lunch) and still benefit. Purchase a journal and take some time every day to write. Not only will it relieve negative feelings but you'll have a permanent record of your thoughts.

Hypnosis   A review of studies provided evidence that self-hypnosis combined with targeted imagery enhanced mood. Six weeks of training almost halved recurrence of depression, improved mood, and reduced levels of clinical depression and anxiety. See Menstrual Bleeding for more information.

■ Dizziness

Avoid:
Inactivity

Focus On:
Qigong   Qigong is a simple and effective exercise popular in China. If done persistently, it helps make you stronger, more balanced, energetic, and healthy. It has special curative effects on the digestive, respiratory, circulatory, and nervous systems. There are standing, sitting, and walking forms of the exercise. For more information consult *The Wonders of Qigong*, Wayfarer Publications, Los Angeles.

1. Stand with toes of both feet turned inward. Rest your weight on the balls of your feet, knees straight, chest expanded, abdomen pulled in, and eyes closed. Focus your breathing on a spot just below your navel. Keep the tip of your tongue against the hard palate (roof of mouth) while inhaling and return it to normal while exhaling. Count 15 inhales and exhales before proceeding to step 2.

2. Extend both arms straight ahead at shoulder level, palms face out and fingers face up as though pushing against a wall. Count 10 inhales and exhales.

3. Extend both arms straight out to the side. Count 15 inhales and exhales.

4. Extend both arms backward, palms face downward, and fingers close together. Press your arms against your ribs and let your chest incline forward about 30 degrees. Count 15 inhales and exhales.

5. Gradually add a couple of breaths to each movement up to 100 total inhales and exhales.

■ Fatigue

Avoid:
Body Tension

Focus On:
Hypnosis   Self-hypnosis training has been reported to reduce fatigue, enhance vigor, and reduce confusion. Get your body relaxed then picture yourself energized and strong. For more information See Menstrual Bleeding section.

■ Hair Loss/Thinning

Avoid:
Negative Thinking About Your Hair

Focus On:
Guided Imagery   Get into a relaxed position and picture the circulation increasing in your scalp. Picture your hair thickening and strengthening.

■ Headaches

Avoid:
Tension   Meditation, imagery, and yoga all have strong research support for reducing tension and headaches. Here are some approaches to try.

Focus On:
Yoga

Child Pose
1. Kneel with your feet behind you and sit on your heels, keeping the top of your feet flat on the floor.
2. Bend forward slowly until your forehead rests on the floor or on folded towels.
3. Clasp your hands behind your back.
4. Breathe regularly for a couple of minutes, relaxing into the position.

Neck Roll
Don't do this exercise if you have whiplash, disk disease, or any problem in the cervical (neck) spine.

1. Sit in a comfortable position, relaxing your shoulders, arms, and hands.
2. Breathe regularly, letting your breath move toward your center, focusing on your navel.
3. Slowly turn your head to the right as far as you can comfortably go. Picture yourself going an inch or so farther, then return your head to the center.
4. Repeat, turning your head to the left and picturing yourself turning an inch or so farther.
5. Let your head drop toward your chest while continuing to breathe. Go only as far as you can comfortably go, then return to the beginning position.
6. Let your head drop back and look up at the sky, letting your chin move up as far as you can comfortably go while continuing to breathe.
7. Repeat, looking left, right, up, and down, noticing increased flexibility with each try.

Stress-Release Exercises While sitting in a chair, complete these exercises every hour to relieve stress in your shoulders, neck, upper arms, and back.

1. Round your shoulders forward three times and back three times.
2. Press your shoulders down three times.
3. Push your shoulders up three times.
4. Look up and look down three times.
5. Lean forward and let your head and hands dangle toward the floor for a few slow breaths or until you're ready to sit up.

Reflexology The theory behind reflexology, an ancient Chinese therapy, is that every point on the body is linked to a reference or *re-*

flex point on the foot, ear, or hand. The foot is often used because of its sensitivity. Each foot houses thousands of nerve endings, which according to reflex theory are connected to organs, bones, glands, and muscles throughout the body. The idea is to stimulate these reflex points. The reflex points corresponding to headaches and sinus problems are found at the tips and sides of the toes and the sides of both feet.

Remove your shoes and socks. If your feet are soiled, wash them. If your feet are dry, apply some moisturizing cream or olive oil, and find a comfortable spot to sit. Follow the directions below to work some of the tension out of your head and neck.

1. Hold one foot with one hand. With your other hand start at the edge of your heel and press your thumb into the bottom of your foot using enough pressure to cause a "good hurt."
2. Work your thumb up every inch of your foot, working toward your toes.
3. Work the top of your foot using your thumb and fingers to walk along the surface.
4. Spend extra time in tender areas.
5. Work up the back, across the top, and down the front of each toe to its base.
6. Work in the webbing of each toe.
7. Work above the nail line of each toe.
8. Pull out each toe and circle it around clockwise and then counterclockwise.

■ Heart Disease

Avoid:
Pushing Yourself to the Limit

Focus On:
Imagery Practice picturing yourself relaxing. In one study, imagery produced a significant reduction in worry and stress.

Touch Therapy Therapeutic touch can help calm you down. A study of 150 adults showed that therapeutic touch reduced worry in participants significantly over traditional treatment.

Qigong After 10 weeks of performing qigong, blood pressure decreased significantly. Levels of stress hormones (norepinephrine, epinephrine, cortisol) and stress level were also significantly reduced. The results suggest that qigong reduces blood pressure by stabilizing the nervous system. For specific qigong exercises, see the Dizziness section.

■ Hot Flashes

Avoid:
Stressing Yourself Stress reduction measures such as abdominal breathing, relaxation therapy, self-hypnosis, and guided imagery may be helpful in decreasing the vasomotor flushing called hot flashes.

Focus On:
Relaxation Training In one study of women who participated in applied relaxation training, the number of hot flashes decreased and continued to decrease at a 6-month follow-up.

Hypnosis After using self-hypnosis, the number, duration, and severity of hot flashes were significantly reduced for 10 healthy volunteers and 4 women diagnosed with breast cancer. To reduce hot flashes, relax your body totally and picture it staying cool and calm. See Menstrual Bleeding for more information.

■ Insomnia/Sleep Problems

Avoid:
Negative Thoughts About Sleep

Focus On:
Cognitive-Behavioral Treatments Cognitive-behavioral treatments for insomnia and sleep problems have been shown to be effective. This kind of approach includes examining and changing automatic thoughts and assumptions (e.g., "I can't sleep" or "I'll never get to sleep"), learning new and more positive ways of setting the stage for sleep, changing behaviors to effect better coping, and learning new behaviors/responses (telling yourself, "I can go to sleep; all I have to do is close my eyes, and my body will start to relax").

Hypnosis In one study of healthy volunteers and women diagnosed with breast cancer, participants reported better sleep and less insomnia after four weekly 1-hour sessions learning to practice hypnosis. To use hypnosis for sleep, get into a relaxed state (use a relaxation tape if necessary) and tell yourself you're going to keep your eyes open no matter how heavy your eyelids become. Feel your eyelids getting heavier and heavier. Use repetitive phrases in a monotone voice for the best results. See Menstrual Bleeding section for more information.

■ Itchiness

Avoid:
Negative Thoughts About Comfort

Focus On:
Hypnosis Hypnosis can improve or resolve numerous skin issues that lead to itching. It has been shown especially cost-effective for conditions unresponsive to standard medical treatments. Suggestions that may reduce itching once a relaxed state is attained include: *Not for me, but for my body, this itch is damaging. It means my body is out of balance. To live comfortably, I need my body in balance. To the point I wish to live in comfort, I will itch when I choose to and at the body location I choose.*

■ Joint and Muscle Pain

Avoid:
Negative Thoughts About Pain

Focus On:
Hypnosis Hypnosis was significantly more effective for relieving pain than minimal treatment or the use of an occlusion appliance with regard to women's report of facial pain. The researchers in the study concluded that hypnosis was an effective treatment for pain, especially for subjective pain parameters. See Menstrual Bleeding for more information.

■ Memory Loss and Foggy Thinking

Avoid:
Shallow Breathing and Worrying

Focus On:
Deep Breathing When you're stressed, you start breathing in the upper part of your chest, cutting off a sufficient supply of oxygen. Deep breathing can restore the balance, slow you down, and help your memory. Find a quiet spot and relax your body, letting your breathing move to your abdominal area—your center.

Imagery If you lost a key or can't find something, picture what you were doing the last time you saw that item. If you relax and wait, the location will often pop into your mind.

Unswitching According to Dr. David Williams, a holistic physician, if you bump into things, drop things, can't concentrate, and have trouble remembering things, you could be "switched." Here's how he explains what happens. Energy moves through your body by way of a meridian (acupuncture/acupressure) system that follows well-defined directions and pathways. Stress can cause a pattern to switch or flow in the wrong direction. Fatigue, allergies, nervousness, worry, and poor diet are just a few situations that can lead to switching.

1. Locate the acupuncture point named K-27 (Kidney-27) on the front of your body where the first rib, collarbone, and breastbone come together. Place your fingers on either side of your collarbone and slowly follow it toward the center of your chest to a small depression or hole where the three bones come together. This is K-27.
2. Place the index and middle finger of one hand on either side of your belly button.
3. Place the index finger of your other hand on K-27 on the right.

4. At the same time, gently rub in both areas in a rotary fashion for 15–20 seconds.

5. Move your top index finger to the left K-27 point and rub both spots again for 15–20 seconds.

■ Menstrual Bleeding

Avoid:

Situations Evoking Tension Feeling tense, out of control, and pressured can interfere with healthy body functioning.

Focus On:

Hypnosis Hypnosis is useful for stopping excess bleeding. It decreases the frequency and severity of bleeding episodes. It also provides increased feelings of control and confidence, during which positive suggestions are given. Hypnosis is really self-hypnosis because no one accepts a suggestion unless he or she wants to.

Hypnosis is really just an enhanced sense of relaxation and focus. You can consult a hypnotist or learn the technique by listening to hypnosis tapes. Try the following exercise to see if hypnosis is for you:

1. Sit or lie in a comfortable position. Remind yourself that whenever you want to come out of hypnosis you can.

2. Focus on a candle, picture, crack in the ceiling, or some other object to encourage eye fixation.

3. While watching the object, suggest your eyes are getting heavier—they're starting to sting or beginning to flutter. Use whichever feeling works best to induce eyelid heaviness.

4. Preselect a word or phrase to use as a suggestion, which is to be used the moment your eyes close. The words *relax now* or a color or a place that is beautiful and has special meaning to you can be used.

5. Relax all your muscles. While keeping your eyes closed, start with your forearms and biceps. First tighten, then release them until your arms feel relaxed. Move to your face. Tighten and release several times until your face feels relaxed. Repeat the same procedure with your neck, shoulders, chest, stomach, lower back, buttocks, thighs, calves, and toes until your entire body is relaxed.

6. Begin to notice a heavy feeling in your arm. Notice your arm getting lighter and lighter as if balloons were tied to it, lifting it higher and higher. Soon your hand will begin to move, imperceptibly at first, but then it will float, moving closer and closer to your face. When your hand touches your face, you will be in hypnosis.

7. When you're ready, tell yourself it's time to return from hypnosis. You can also tell yourself before you get into a relaxed state that you will open your eyes in __ minutes. Either way you will feel refreshed and relaxed.

■ Osteoporosis

Avoid:
Negative Thinking About Bone Growth

Focus On:
Hypnosis   A study of bone healing provided evidence that hypnosis not only increased bone growth as judged by radiographic and orthopedic assessment but also increased mobility and lowered the use of pain medicine. See Menstrual Bleeding section for more information.

■ Sex Drive Reduction and Intercourse Discomfort

Avoid:
Negative Thinking About Intercourse

Focus On:
Hypnotic Desensitization   Fear and anxiety are of tremendous import in the production and maintenance of a symptom. Vaginal spasms that prevent intercourse can be effectively treated by systematic desensitization. The first part of the treatment is to imagine an anxiety hierarchy (see the 10 steps below) of increasingly erotic and sexually intimate situations, which will later be reproduced with the partner, until sexual intercourse is achieved.

The last step in the hierarchy is penetration. The first step might be thinking about having sex. If this is the case, write down those steps and the steps in between.

Lola, a 51-year-old second-grade teacher, worked with me to develop a hierarchy. Here's the one she used:

1. Think about making love.
2. Prepare to make love.
3. Lie down on the bed with my husband.
4. Kiss my husband.
5. Remove my clothes.
6. Feel his hands rubbing my body.
7. Watch him remove his clothes.
8. Feel his erection against me.
9. Oil my vagina.
10. Guide his penis into my vagina.

Once you have your hierarchy developed, purchase a relaxation tape or take a relaxation class until you can relax all the muscles in your body at will. Imagine the first step in your hierarchy. If you still feel calm, imagine the second step in your hierarchy. Whenever you begin to feel anxious, listen to the relaxation tape or stop thinking of your hierarchy and focus on relaxing your body until you feel totally at ease. (You can't be anxious and have a relaxed body—it's impossible!)

Work back and forth between your hierarchy and relaxing your body until you can move through all the steps (from the least anxiety-provoking number 1 to the most anxiety-provoking number 10). When you can move through all the steps in your imagination and remain calm, you are ready to try it out with your partner.

Make sure you talk to your partner about the process so that you both know how to proceed. Also get your partner's support. Since this process will enhance your lovemaking, tell your partner that, too. If you experience any anxiety, stop making love, turn on the tape, or use a relaxation exercise to relax your body. When you're ready, resume lovemaking.

■ Skin Problems

Avoid:
Negative Thinking About Safety

Focus On:
Hypnosis   Skin is a living, breathing organ. Hypnosis has been used effectively to bring nourishment to the skin. Suggestions to use once total relaxation has been achieved include: *I feel safe to be me,* and *I lovingly protect myself with healthy skin.*

■ Urinary Symptoms

Avoid:
Negative Thinking About Bladder Control

Focus On:
Affirmations Choose one of the following suggestions and either say or write the idea many times a day:

- I have power over my body. I can tell my bladder when it needs to empty and when not to bother me. I declare myself in charge of my body.
- My bladder is toning and strengthening. I will no longer feel strong urges that force me to urinate even though my bladder is not yet full. But I will now receive urges to empty my bladder when it is properly full.

■ Weight Gain

Avoid:
Negative Thinking About Weight Control

Focus On:
Hypnosis Hypnosis can help with weight loss. At least one study provided evidence that hypnotherapy focused on stress reuction allowed for significant weight loss that still was effective 18 months after treatment. Get yourself into a relaxed state using a relaxation or self-hypnosis tape if necessary and give yourself the suggestion to stay calm and lose weight. If necessary, have a session or two with a hypnotherapist. See Menstrual Bleeding for more information.

Relationships

Katrina, a 38-year-old mother of twins, underwent a hysterectomy, throwing her body into menopause. When she and her
husband, Doug, came to see me, Katrina said hot flashes, vaginal
dryness, and headaches interfered with lovemaking. Her husband
reported feeling left out and clueless about what to do to make
things better. I gave them a checklist to help identify their communication styles. We practiced empathy and assertiveness skills, and I
showed them how to paraphrase each other's comments to make
sure they understood each other. They also practiced telling what
was positive about their lovemaking and the changes they desired.

Your body changes rapidly during menopause. Research has provided evidence that having a good relationship with your partner, a
positive mood, and keeping yourself healthy with exercise and other
positive lifestyle behaviors leads to greater life satisfaction. To enhance your relationship with your partner, you must communicate
clearly about the changes you're undergoing and what might help.
Talking things out, giving your partner tips about what is helpful,

and making the appropriate adjustments will help your menopause experience be more positive. This chapter provides specific ways to do just that!

My Communication Patterns

Check off the statements that best describe how you communicate and wish to be communicated with:

❑   1. I like to make the big decisions around the house.
❑   2. I like to make the small decisions around the house.
❑   3. I think we should discuss the big decisions and decide them together.
❑   4. I think we both should be involved in small household decisions.
❑   5. It's important for me to discuss things; it helps me feel closer to you.
❑   6. If you come to me with a problem, I expect to solve it.
❑   7. When I'm angry, I don't talk.
❑   8. When I'm afraid, I get angry.
❑   9. It takes me a while to get in touch with my feelings.
❑ 10. When I am pushed to talk, I won't.
❑ 11. When I'm embarrassed, I blush or disappear.
❑ 12. When I'm embarrassed, I get angry.

Katrina revealed that she liked to discuss issues with Doug because that made her feel closer to him. He said when Katrina brought up an issue, he thought that meant she wanted him to solve it. Katrina complained that Doug didn't answer right away when she asked him what his feelings were, and he said she pressured him. Both Katrina and Doug said they felt embarrassed about discussing their sexual activity.

Ask your partner to complete the checklist, too. Your answers (and your partner's) should give you some information you may not have had before. Knowing more about what makes the other person uncomfortable can be very helpful. This will be a good start and help you better understand your partner. If you're not doing so already, establish a weekly time to work on establishing better communication habits. Read on for more ideas.

■ Features of Good Communication

Assertiveness and empathy are two skills you and your partner both need.

Assertiveness vs. Aggressiveness or Avoidance

Assertive communication clearly states goals, needs, and expectations. The speaker takes responsibility for the words by using "I" messages ("I want to talk with you about . . ." or "I feel disappointed we aren't making love" or "I apologize" or "I would like to . . .").

Passive or passive-aggressive communication occurs when you don't directly express your thoughts, feelings, or wishes. You may communicate one message with your body and facial expressions or discount your opinions or keep them to yourself. You tend to let the other person control the conversation but may use zingers (passive-aggressive) to retaliate or express your displeasure with the other person. Blaming messages are also passive-aggressive ("You're wrong" or "I feel you ought to change" or "I want you to . . .").

Avoiding communication occurs when you don't bring up your needs or desires, or you change the subject when your partner does. Read the examples below that show how Katrina progressed from avoidance to passive-aggressiveness to assertiveness.

Communication Example 1

Doug: "What's this 'My Communication Patterns' thing?"

Katrina: "Nothing. Don't worry about it. Sorry I bothered you." (Avoidance)

After additional coaching, Doug and Katrina tried again.

Communication Example 2

Doug: "What am I supposed to do with this 'My Communication Patterns' thing?"

Katrina: (Looking at me) "See what I have to put up with?" (Passive-aggressive)

After more discussion, Katrina and Doug tried again.

Doug: "Where do you get these things? Every week it's some new thing you want to try."

Katrina: "I guess it seems that way, but I'm asking you to bear with me and fill out this form. I think it can help us understand each other better." (Assertive)

We started to discuss types of assertive responses Katrina and Doug could use to help keep the conversation on track should it go awry. They appear below.

Assertive Probing Criticism is often used by others to avoid important feelings or wishes. Assertive probing assists in determining whether criticism is constructive or manipulative and clarifies unclear comments. Focus on the part of the criticism that's most bothersome. In the case above, Katrina could have asked Doug, "What is it that bothers you about me asking you to try new things?"

Content-to-Process Shift When the focus or point of the conversation drifts away from the original topic, use the content-to-process shift to bring you back to an important point. You could say, "Let's go back to what we were discussing" or "Let's not argue. We were discussing . . ."

Momentary Delay If you're feeling overwhelmed, you can delay a discussion to a later time. Some comments to use are "Let me think about what you said and let's talk about it after dinner" or "I need more time to decide. I'll get back to you tomorrow."

Assertiveness Tips While practicing assertiveness, use the following rules:

- Speak up and share your goals, needs, or limits (saying no is a legitimate and assertive response when you're feeling overwhelmed and overstressed). You could say something like, "I'd like to talk with you about household tasks. Is this a good time?" or "I'm feeling stressed and I need your help" or "I don't really want advice; I just want to blow off some steam" or "No, I can't take on any more work."
- Treat your partner with respect and dignity. Provide gentle reminders—for example, "I'd really like to tell you more about what's going on with me."
- If you lose your temper, reschedule your conversation when both of you have cooled down.
- Start with a positive comment such as "I really appreciate you." (A nice hug wouldn't hurt, either. Loving touch can enhance closeness, so communication barriers drop away.)
- Be as specific as you can, identifying your goals and wishes.
- Use "I" messages that contain *when* ("When we have plans to spend time together . . ."), *I feel* ("I feel disappointed . . .") *because* ("Because I've been looking forward to being with you").
- Let your partner know that you're in this together and that you're willing to negotiate—for example, "I'll do this for you if you do _____ for me."
- Ask your partner what was heard and restate what you meant if necessary so you know you've been understood.

Empathy

Empathy is the ability to accurately perceive the feelings and perceptions of other people. You temporarily put aside your own needs and make every effort to understand your partner. The result is a partner who feels heard, validated, and cared for. When this happens, you're more likely to find a positive solution to the problem.

The best way to improve your ability to be empathic is to listen to your partner talk, then paraphrase back what you hear. Look at the examples below of Katrina and Doug's beginning efforts at empathy.

Low Empathy

Katrina: "Will you fill this out?" (Hands him a copy of "My Communication Patterns.")

Doug: "I don't have time for this!"

Katrina: "You never do anything I ask."

Doug: "Now what—are you going to start crying again?"

We discussed the results. Neither Katrina nor Doug were satisfied with the outcome. We talked about paraphrasing and how to reflect back what your partner says as a way to enhance communication.

Beginning Empathy

After a few sessions, Katrina started to convey a more accurate awareness of her partner's feelings.

Katrina: "I just filled out a communication list. I'd like you to help me out and fill one out, too." (Hands him the form.)

Doug: (Looks at the list and sets it down.) "What is this? You think I don't know how to talk?"

Katrina: "Is that how it seems to you?" (Asks for more information.)

Doug: "Yeah, you come in here, telling me to fill out some list."

Katrina: "You're feeling pressured by me?" (Reflects partner's reaction.)

Doug: "Sure, wouldn't you?"

Katrina: "I don't want to pressure you. It's important to me to know how you feel."

Doug: (Picks up the list.) "All right, if it means that much to you, I'll do it."

To increase your empathy skills, interview your partner as if you're a reporter for the local newspaper. Find out how your partner feels about and sees a situation. Take your time and approach this exercise seriously. Write everything down and check to see that you are using the following empathy rules:

- Maintain good eye contact.
- Listen to whatever your partner has to say without interrupting, feeling helpless, or getting angry.
- Ask "how" and "what" questions to help you understand your partner's feelings and thoughts.
- Restate what you mean if your partner doesn't understand you. (Be sure to check and ask what your partner heard.)
- Avoid "why" questions (e.g., "Why did you do that?" or "Why would you do that?"). Why questions increase defensiveness and stall communication.
- Avoid making assumptions. Verify your impressions by checking out what you think you heard—for example, "Here's what I heard you say. Is that what you meant?"
- Use "I" statements to own your feelings and thoughts—for example, "I feel angry" or "I'd like to . . ."
- Avoid being judgmental or critical. Both block communication.
- Find areas of agreement. Compromise is part of making a relationship better. Whenever two or more people are involved, there's bound to be some disagreement. It's healthy, but so is working out compromises. Use your negotiation skills. You can promise to fulfill one of your partner's wishes in exchange for your partner fulfilling one of yours. You'll both get something you want. That's the benefit of a compromise.

■ Telling Your Partner About Your Menopause Changes

Although you may be in the throes of menopause, remember that your partner has no clue what you're going through. It's up to you to tell your partner what is happening, what to expect, and how to help. Choose a quiet time when the TV isn't blaring and neither of you is stressed. You may want to use the suggestions below (as they are or in a modified form) to tell your partner about the specific menopause changes you're having. Start with a positive comment showing you appreciate your partner.

Breast Cancer and Other Cancers

"I remember how good you were with your mother when she had a mastectomy. My chances of developing breast cancer have increased because of menopause. That scares me, so I'm planning to take action to prevent me from getting cancer by eating more fruits and vegetables, fish, and soy. I'm going off coffee and starting to drink red clover tea. I've also been learning to use imagery to picture my breasts healthy, and I've started an exercise program. I'd really like you to join me. What about a short walk after dinner?"

Cold Hands

"I want to thank you for not disturbing me when I was working on my report. I've been suffering from cold hands for a while now, and I'll be using a relaxation tape to increase circulation. I'll put a DO NOT DISTURB sign on the bedroom door when I'm relaxing, and I'd appreciate it if you didn't enter at that time. It might also help if you massage my hands when you have time and I'll massage your feet in return."

Depression, Nervousness, and Irritability

"I want to let you know how much I appreciate you being so patient with my moods lately. There are some jokes about menopause making women crazy. My personality isn't changing, but there are definite chemical reactions inside me that can bring on mood swings. I know the way I've been acting may be confusing for you. I'm taking some herbs and planning to start an exercise program to lift my mood. Here's another thing I can suggest. I'll give you a time-out sign when I want to be left alone. When the mood passes, I'll come and find you."

Dizziness

"I wanted to thank you for watching the kids when I wasn't feeling good yesterday. I also wanted to share some information with you. My nurse practitioner says I'm low on iron and that's why I've been having dizzy spells. I bought some iron pots to cook in and more foods that contain iron for us to eat. In the meantime, if you notice me having trouble walking, keep an eye on me. I'm going to be doing some exercises with a ball and I'll need you to play catch with me, if that's okay with you."

Fatigue

"I appreciated that you let me sleep late this morning. I've been a lot more tired since menopause started. Part of it is the hot flashes I'm having that make it difficult for me to sleep. That's why I've been waking up tired. I'd like to sit down with you and set up a schedule so that you can help me with the household tasks. I just don't have the energy to do it all at this time. In return, I'll _____ the way you've told me you'd like me to."

Hair Loss/Thinning

"Thanks for not giving me a hard time about all the hair I've been leaving in the shower and on the bathroom floor. I'm really upset about how much hair I've been losing. It's due to menopause. I've decided to use henna on my hair rather than dye it like I used to. I read it's safer and will thicken my hair. I'm doing a few other things like eating food and taking herbs that strengthen my hair."

Headaches

"Did I tell you I appreciate you today? I do, and because I do, there's something I want to share with you. I've been having a lot more headaches since menopause changes started. I've signed up for an exercise program at the gym, and my nurse practitioner showed me how to use imagery to turn the pain into a color, then into a liquid, and let it flow out of me. That works pretty well. You might consider using it for your _____ " (headaches, tennis elbow, or whatever pain or discomfort your partner suffers from).

Heart Disease

"I know how much you helped your dad when he had his heart attack. Heart disease is the number one cause of death in women after menopause. Because I don't want to develop heart disease, I'd like us to take a walk after dinner every evening, and I'll be serving more vegetables and fruits that protect the heart. I'm asking for your cooperation with this."

Hot Flashes

"I appreciate that you didn't give me a bad time last night when I had so many hot flashes. Although each flash only lasts a few minutes, they're very uncomfortable. I've been getting them a lot at night, so I'm putting a fan by my side of the bed and I'll probably be kicking off the covers and not sleeping very well. It would help if you remind me to dress for the hot flashes so I can take off a layer or two if they start. Stress can bring them on, so let's try not to argue."

Insomnia/Sleep Problems

"I appreciate that you didn't bug me about waking you up a couple of times last night. I've been having trouble sleeping since menopause started. It would help if you reminded me to take my calcium and B vitamins before bedtime. Maybe we could massage each other's feet as a way to relax before bedtime."

Itchiness

"I wanted to thank you for helping me with the groceries yesterday, and I'd like to talk to you about something. I've been having some itchy, crawling feelings that I think are related to menopause. I put lotion where I can reach, but I could use help putting some on my back. Fish oil is supposed to help, so we'll be eating more tuna and Spanish mackerel, too. Maybe you can help keep me from getting dehydrated by reminding me to drink more water."

Joint and Muscle Pain

"Remember when your mom had arthritis so bad? You were a big help to her, and I'm going to need your help now. I have joint and muscle pains like I never had before menopause started. I'm taking more calcium and magnesium, but I also need to eat more seafood and green leafy veggies. Those foods are good for you, too, so I'll be planning more meals around them if that's okay with you."

Memory Loss and Foggy Thinking

"I really appreciate the way you've been helping me lately. I hope it's okay to ask for a little more help. Since I stopped menstruating regularly, I've been having trouble remembering things. If you see me put my keys somewhere or see my things where they don't belong, I'd appreciate it if you'd tell me where you see them. I'm off alcohol and caffeine. I'll only be drinking green tea because that's what will help my memory. I'm also getting off the low-carb diet we've been on together because dieting is bad for the memory. You're going to be seeing more whole-grain cereals and breads around, too, because they're good for memory. I bought a reverse osmosis water filter system to make sure toxins in our drinking water aren't contributing to my memory problem."

Menstrual Bleeding

"You were so helpful buying me mulch for my garden and I wanted to thank you for that. I also wanted to talk to you about something that's happening with me. My menstrual bleeding is getting heavier and more unpredictable. I need you to be patient with me during these times. I'll let you know when they are. I'm also going to stop eating red meat and dairy products because they may increase my bleeding. I'll be eating more fruits, veggies, prunes, raisins, and wheat germ and cooking with turmeric. Easy exercise will also help. I'd like us to start taking a slow bike ride together after dinner. What do you say?"

Osteoporosis

"I wanted to tell you how much I appreciate you and to ask for your help. My risk for bone loss and bone fractures just went up because of menopause, so I'm off sodas, animal protein, sugar, salt, caffeine, and alcohol—all things that weaken bones. I bought a bottle of B vitamins. They're good for reducing my risk for bone fractures and help with mood, too. I also bought a bottle of calcium citrate, and I'll be serving more sardines, salmon, shrimp, soy foods, onions, and dark green leafy veggies because they have calcium that strengthens bone. I won't be keeping the coffee pot on, either, because I'll be drinking red clover tea or water to reduce bone loss. I just found out smoking increases my risk of osteoporosis, so I've signed up for a Stop Smoking course at the Lung Association on Wednesdays after work. Maybe you can pick up some Chinese takeout that night on your way home unless you want to cook. I also picked up a brochure at the Adult Center. They're offering two classes that could help me: yoga and ballroom dance. I thought we could go together."

Sex Drive Reduction and Intercourse Discomfort

Be aware that men go through their own set of doubts in middle age. They often report a decline in sexual activity after age 50. They may take longer to reach ejaculation, lose erections, or not be able to reach climax. Many men fear they will fail sexually as they get older. Be understanding, and don't make a big deal about climaxes. Tell your partner you want to share a pleasurable time together and that a climax would be a dividend, but it isn't necessary. A hug and a whisper about your continued love can enhance your relationship even more.

Other comments you might wish to express include: "I want to thank you for being patient with me about lovemaking. My vagina has gotten smaller due to menopause. That's probably why I've been uncomfortable making love. I found some things that could help to make lovemaking better, and I'm asking for your cooperation. I'll be eating more alfalfa sprouts, dried beans, apples, seeds, soy foods, and oat cereal to strengthen my vagina. I also bought an herbal capsule that contains black cohosh, dong quai, ginkgo, and damiana to enhance sexual desire and keep me from having hot flashes during lovemaking. I talked to my nurse practitioner. She's weaning me off the Zoloft I've been taking for depression, and I'll be making my way through a book called *Feeling Good* and doing the depression reduction exercise. I'd like us to start having regular sex again because that's the best way to keep my vagina healthy. I'm going to try using castor oil, vitamin E, and olive oil to lubricate my vagina before insertion. I'd like us to have more foreplay and maybe focus on me having an orgasm first so then I can concentrate on what pleasures you. I've written down a couple of things you do that turn me on when we're making love. I'd like you to do them more often—for example, massaging my feet and thighs as part of foreplay. Why don't you give me a list of things that turn you on and I'll be sure to do them?"

If you've never talked this openly before, now is the time to start.

Remember: your partner can't know what pleases you unless you verbalize it.

If penetration is painful, having your orgasm *before* penetration will be helpful because orgasm increases circulation, making your vagina more ready for entry. Try keeping your legs flat on the bed at first so penetration isn't so deep. You can also put your hands on your pubic bone to control the depth, frequency, and force of penetration. That can decrease discomfort; so can being on top, where you can control timing and depth of penetration. Picturing your vagina moistening and lubricating can work, too. Discuss this issue with your partner—for example, "I'd like to try having my orgasm first, *before* penetration. That way I can give my full attention to pleasuring you."

Skin Problems

"I want to thank you for doing the grocery shopping yesterday and let you know why I'm serving more eggs, poultry, fish, soybeans, and whole grains. These foods can keep my skin healthy and wrinkle-free. I bought a calendula lotion and put it in the bathroom cabinet. It's for itchy, scaling skin, so if you want to use it, too, go ahead. I'm also using pine tar soap for my skin. It's the brown bar in the shower, and you can use it if you have any skin problems. I bought some 2-pound weights because I read that pushing and pulling during weight lifting tightens up the face and prevents facial wrinkles. If you see me making strange faces, it's just me doing my face-firming exercises." You could also add that you want to look youthful to please your partner.

Urinary Symptoms

"I really appreciate that you stopped at so many rest rooms for me on our trip yesterday. Menopause has increased my urge to urinate, and I can get bladder infections more often. To stop that from happening, I'm taking an herb called corn silk and drinking nettle tea. I've also replaced our aluminum cookware with iron pots and pans because aluminum can irritate the bladder. I want to buy a reverse osmosis water filtration system, too, to make sure I'm not getting any toxic metals that can cause urinary problems."

Weight Gain

"I want to thank you for reminding me that I'm gaining weight. I didn't want to hear it at first, but we did agree to remind each other, and I do want to look sexy for you. I know you think I should go on a diet, but all the research says that's a bad idea, and even if I did lose weight, I wouldn't keep it off. Instead, I've decided to just eat smaller dinners, eat a nutritious breakfast, and eat small meals throughout the day. I found a hypnotist who's had a lot of success with helping women gain confidence that they can take off weight and keep it off. I'm also asking for your cooperation. Please don't put any junk food in the refrigerator or cabinets. If it's not around, I won't eat it."

PART III

Creating Your Menopause Plan

10

Changes, Demands, and Supports

To create your Living Well with Menopause Plan, begin by identifying the changes, demands, and supports that may be affecting you. The first step in this process is to fill in your Menopause Wellness Profile. This profile will help you identify your menopause changes. You will be using this profile to develop your plan, so take sufficient time to make sure you consider each item.

Rate the severity of all changes you've encountered. In the case of risks, rate your reaction to knowing each risk you face.

Menopause Wellness Profile

	Doesn't Affect Me Much If at All	This Is a Real Problem, but I Can Function	I Can Barely Function with This/Thinking About This
1. Breast cancer and other cancers	_____	_____	_____
2. Cold hands	_____	_____	_____
3. Depression, nervousness, and irritability	_____	_____	_____
4. Dizziness	_____	_____	_____
5. Fatigue	_____	_____	_____
6. Hair loss/thinning	_____	_____	_____
7. Headaches	_____	_____	_____
8. Heart disease	_____	_____	_____
9. Hot flashes	_____	_____	_____
10. Insomnia/sleep problems	_____	_____	_____
11. Itchiness	_____	_____	_____
12. Joint and muscle pain	_____	_____	_____
13. Memory loss and foggy thinking	_____	_____	_____
14. Bleeding (irregular or heavy)	_____	_____	_____
15. Osteoporosis	_____	_____	_____
16. Sex drive reduction and intercourse discomfort	_____	_____	_____
17. Skin Problems	_____	_____	_____
18. Urinary symptoms	_____	_____	_____
19. Weight gain	_____	_____	_____

■ Changes and Demands

The changes you're undergoing are only one part of what can hamper you. They use up your energy; the more changes you face, the less energy you have to make your menopause a positive process. Check yes or no next to each change to see where you stand.

1. Being treated for a serious or chronic condition ☐ yes ☐ no
2. Raising children ☐ yes ☐ no
3. Empty nest reaction ☐ yes ☐ no
4. Change in a relationship ☐ yes ☐ no
5. Change in workload ☐ yes ☐ no
6. Change in job security ☐ yes ☐ no
7. Dieting ☐ yes ☐ no
8. Change in self-image ☐ yes ☐ no
9. Loss of friend or family member ☐ yes ☐ no
10. Addition to the family ☐ yes ☐ no
11. Marriage ☐ yes ☐ no
12. Family tensions ☐ yes ☐ no
13. Separation/divorce ☐ yes ☐ no
14. Moving to new residence ☐ yes ☐ no
15. Vacation ☐ yes ☐ no
16. Natural disaster ☐ yes ☐ no
17. Remodeling ☐ yes ☐ no
18. Other demands (please list)
19. Other changes (please list)

Supports

If you have sufficient supports, your menopause process may proceed positively. Complete the checklist to take an inventory of your supports.

_____ 1. My partner listens to me and is supportive of me.

_____ 2. My partner helps out with household tasks.

_____ 3. My children support me.

_____ 4. My children help out around the house.

_____ 5. My parents are supportive of me.

_____ 6. One or both of my parents help out when needed.

_____ 7. I have at least one supportive friend.

_____ 8. I have at least one friend who helps out when needed.

_____ 9. I have a health care practitioner who listens to me, explains whatever I don't understand, and is willing to consider alternative and complementary procedures.

_____ 10. I belong to a support group of menopausal women that provides support and understanding, information about available resources, reduced feelings of isolation, good ideas for solving common problems, hope and optimism, and a potential for new friends with common issues. The members are not overly critical or negative, and they do not dominate the discussion.

If you don't have enough supports, consider joining a support group, teaching your family empathy and supportive skills, finding a more supportive health practitioner (see the next chapter), or finding a new friend who's working on the same issues you are and who's supportive.

11

Finding and Working with the Right Practitioner

Much of having a positive menopause involves self-care. If you face a hysterectomy, endometriosis, or other complications, you will need a supportive practitioner. There are no menopause specialists, although maybe there should be, but there are practitioners who can look at the broad spectrum of medical and complementary/alternative approaches.

Since there are no menopause specialty physicians, you will probably start your search with a primary care physician, maybe a general practitioner, internist, or primary care gynecologist. Proper assistance may require endocrine, nutrition, orthopedic, psychological, complementary/holistic, and herbalist care. If you can find a holistically oriented general practitioner, that's even better, because you will receive an integrated approach that includes conventional and alternative therapies, or at least referral to complementary practitioners.

I bumped into Jessica at a local library book signing. This 51-year-old Sunday school teacher told me she was disap-

pointed in her traditional physician, who gave her no time to ask questions about the hormone treatment he had ordered for her menopause changes. She asked me for some ideas. Over tea the next day, we discussed her possibilities, from types of practitioners to deciding if she wanted to switch health care providers.

■ Types of Holistic/Complementary Practitioners

As a holistic/complementary practitioner myself, I believe you should have at least one holistic practitioner on your team because it has been shown that most of the changes you're undergoing or may undergo have been shown to respond to a multifaceted approach. The clients I work with are grateful for my holistic approach that helps them integrate alternative methods into their menopause process.

Constantly changing physicians and specialists will probably not be to your advantage. It is up to you to be responsible, get educated, and learn the keys to a wellness approach to menopause. Some of the practitioners available for you to consider appear below.

Acupressure Practitioners

There are various schools of acupressure, but they all involve the same pathways or meridians used by acupuncturists. *Qi,* or energy, is believed to flow along these pathways, energizing and nourishing the body, mind, and spirit. By using the hands to work these points, tensions are released and the flow of qi is enhanced.

Jin Shin Do practitioners teach clients how to hold specific points and use breathing techniques and visualization to release distressing feelings and address neck, shoulder, back tension/pain, headache, chest problems, menstrual difficulties, pelvic tension, digestive stress, respiratory difficulties, insomnia, joint problems, creative blocks, muscle spasms, stress-related difficulties, cerebal palsy, and even developmental problems. Because it is gentle and the recipient is clothed, Jin Shin Do can provide safe physical touch when physical or sexual abuse has occurred. For more information go to http://www.jinshindo.org.

Jin Shin Jyutsu practitioners also use self-help methods to teach their clients how to place the three middle fingers on safety energy locks in specific sequences, called flows, to restore balance. No massage or manipulation is involved. The practitioner merely holds the lock and waits to feel the rhythmic pulsation in the safety lock indicating balance has been restored. For more information, go to http://www.jinshinjyutsu.com. *Shiatsu* is the Japanese version. The whole hand is used to massage, press, and pull. In some moves, even the feet are used.

Acupuncturists

Acupuncture refers to a family of procedures in Chinese medicine and includes the insertion of thin, solid, usually stainless steel needless at precise anatomic locations, classic acupuncture points, motor points, and areas of tenderness. Needles may be manipulated by hand or through attached electrodes. Various waveforms and intensities of voltage may be used. Needles can be stimulated through *moxabustion* (burning an herb) and cupping (a suctioning of the skin through the application of small jars that create a vacuum) or magnets. Acupuncturists usually learn their specialty at colleges of acupuncture and Oriental medicine (http://www.aaom.org), or through the American Academy of Medical Acupuncture (http://www.medicalacupuncture.org).

Guided Imagery Specialists

Imagery is a natural thought process that uses one or more of the five senses and is usually associated with emotions. Imagery is how your right brain conceptualizes, and it is the bridge between the conscious and subconscious mind. It is simply one way your mind thinks. Just as we all dream, we all use imagery to picture a scene in our mind's eye or play a pleasant memory or song back to us. For nearly 20,000 years, imagery has been an integral ingredient in healing practices, for it is the link to the spiritual level of healing.

Holistic practitioners from many disciplines practice guided imagery. To find certified practitioners, contact the Academy for Guided Imagery at (800) 726-2070 or http://www.academyfor guidedimagery.com.

Herbal Practitioners

Herbology is the study of the science and artful use of healing plants or herbs. Every culture has at some point used healing plants as the basis for its medicine. Modern American medicine has its roots in the use of herbs. Until 50 years ago, nearly all entries in the pharmacopeias described herbs. When modern drug research companies began selling synthetic medicines, the values of botanical medicines weren't preserved. Today most of the important herbal research is completed in Europe. While traditional medicine treats organs (heart, mind, lungs, etc.), herbal medicine practitioners recognize that the body is a whole, integrated system greater than the sum of its parts. Herbalists also realize that the whole herb is greater than the sum of its parts. Herbal preparations are only as vital as the quality of the herbs used to prepare them. Herbs are either specifics (used for days or weeks to treat acute conditions) or tonics (used for months to support and nourish body processes).

Since the quality and processing of herbs are not standardized, consult an herbalist who has spent years getting to know the qualities, energies, and properties of herbs so you can be matched to the herbs or combinations that best suit you. To find an herbalist, consult the American Herbalists Guild at http://www.americanherbalists guild.com.

Holistic Nurse Practitioners

Holistic nurse practitioners will not only take a complementary approach to your process but are usually able to prescribe medications should they be needed. They have a master's degree in nursing. More and more nursing programs are providing master's degree programs in holistic nursing. Many nurses with a master's degree in mental health combine a holistic approach with their (primarily) medical basic nursing knowledge. Look for a nurse practitioner who has been board certified as a holistic nurse (HNC), or better yet, as an advanced holistic nurse board-certified (AHN-BC). These initials mean they have demonstrated their ability to work with consumers in a holistic fashion. You can find certified holistic nurses by going to http://www.AHNA.org, e-mailing info@ahna.org, or contacting the American Holistic Nurses Association by phone at (800) 278-2462.

Holistic Physicians

Like holistic nurse practitioners, holistic physicians focus on you as a whole person and how you interact with the environment, not on illness, disease, or specific body parts. A number of medical doctors (MDs) and a larger percentage of osteopaths (DOs) practice holistic medicine and follow holistic principles. You can contact holistic physicians at the American Holistic Medical Associations at http://www.holisticmedicine.org for a free online directory.

Hypnotherapists

Hypnosis is a state of inner focus and a high degree of mental and physical relaxation when you are more open to suggestion. Hypnotic suggestions may consist of direct commands, ideas, and mental imagery to help overcome fears and visualize the successful accomplishment of a goal. The American Society of Clinical Hypnosis provides a list of certified professional hypnotists at http://www.ash.net.

Massage Therapists

There are many kinds of massage. *Neuromuscular therapy (NMT)* is a form of soft-tissue massage including a muscle-by-muscle examination of all soft tissues that may be associated with a particular injury or pain syndrome. NMT addresses the following six factors that create or intensify pain:

1. *Ischemia:* lack of blood and oxygen caused by muscular spasm.
2. *Trigger points:* areas of increased metabolic waste deposits that excite segments of the spinal cord and cause referred pain to other parts of the body.
3. *Nerve entrapment or compression:* pressure on nerves by hard (bone or disk) or soft (muscle, tendon, ligament, fascia, or skin) tissue.
4. *Postural distortion:* The body is held in positions that deviate from an anatomically correct position.
5. *Poor nutrition:* an insufficient intake of necessary nutrients or eating foods that irritate the nervous system.
6. *Emotional upset:* decreased ability to withstand stress.

Swedish massage includes *effleurage* or stroking, *petrissage* or kneading, friction or rubbing, *tapotement* or percussion, and vibration. Skilled practitioners work with a great sensitivity of touch rather than a mechanical routine. Smooth, long, and flowing strokes are performed with palms, finger pads, or forearms, like waves gliding and rippling over the body, bringing fresh blood, oxygen, and nutrients, and taking away waste products. Short and rapid percussive movements include hacking with the outside edge of the hand, tapping with fingertips, cupping or clapping with cupped palms, pummeling with loose or tight fists, and plucking between the thumb and forefinger. Circular linear or transverse strokes made with the thumb, fingertips, palm, or heel of the hand provide friction that spreads muscle fibers and frees muscle from adhesions and scar tissue developed after an injury or surgery. In kneading, the practitioner lifts muscle away from bone, squeezes, rolls, and presses it with both hands, or alternates thumbs in a milking motion that flushes out fluids and metabolic by-products. Practitioners use one hand or the fingertips to create vibration, a rapid, trembling, shaking sensation that stimulates nerves and relaxes tight muscles. The Touch Research Institute at the University of Miami School of Medicine has conducted dozens of clinical trials demonstrating that massage can facilitate growth, increase attentiveness, alleviate pain, improve immune function, and reduce stress.

Find a massage therapist at the American Massage Therapy Association (http://www.amtamassage.org), the Association of Bodywork and Massage Professionals (http://www.healthydoctors.com), or the National Association of Nurse Massage Therapists (http://www.nanmt.org).

Naturopathic Physicians

Naturopathy is a distinct profession of primary health care, emphasizing prevention, treatment, and optimal health using the body's self-healing processes. Doctors of naturopathy (NDs) are general practitioners. The following six principles underlie the practice of naturopathy:

1. There is an inherent self-healing process in you that is ordered and intelligent.
2. Identify and remove the underlying causes of illness rather than just eliminating or suppressing symptoms.
3. The risk of harmful side effects should be minimized.
4. Educate clients, and encourage self-responsibility for health.
5. Treat the whole person.
6. Assess risk factors and encourage prevention.

Naturopaths use many modalities including nutrition, herbs, naturopathic manipulative therapy, counseling, minor surgery, homeopathy, acupuncture, and natural childbirth. Find a naturopath at the Naturopathic Medicine Network (http://www.pandamedicine. com.)

Reflexologists

Reflexology is based on the theory that there are reflex areas in the feet and hands that correspond to all of the glands, organs, and parts of the body. The thumbs and fingers are used to apply specific pressures to these reflex points to relieve stress, improve blood supply, unblock nerve impulses, and help the body rebalance. Clients typically express relief from tension and pain and a heightened sense of well-being and increased energy after a treatment. Because there are 7,200 nerve endings in each foot and each has extensive interconnections through the spinal cord and brain, all areas of the body can be treated by working with the feet.

Some form of reflexology existed in ancient Egypt at least as far back as 2300 B.C., but it was an American, Dr. William H. Fitgerald, who discovered the Chinese method of zone therapy now known as reflexology. To find out more about the procedure and to find reflexology practitioners, go to http://www.reflexology.org.

Relaxation Therapists

Progressive muscle relaxation (PMR) training is a simple and effective form of treatment for helping people learn to relax. The procedure can be used as a primary treatment to complement medical care. It was developed by Dr. Edmund Jacobson in 1929. He discovered that by using a prescribed system of tensing and releasing muscles, deeper levels of relaxation could be reached than by sitting quietly and trying to relax. He based his treatment on the theory that the body responds to anxiety and stress by producing muscle tension, which creates anxiety. He believed that deep muscle relaxation was incompatible with anxiety. The two could not exist at the same time.

In PMR, you are taught to tense and release muscles or muscle groups (e.g., your leg) while being helped to focus on the difference between tension and relaxation. This prepares you to more easily relax your muscles at will. You may even be asked to repeat a phrase such as "I am relaxing." PMR can usually be learned in 1 to 3 weeks if practiced as recommended. There are no cautions, except if the tensing of muscles is overdone, cramping can result. If you're taking a tranquilizer, PMR may enable a decreased dosage. To find a therapist, go to the Directory of Approved Natural Health Practitioners at http://www.nchm.net/DANHP/relax.htm.

Tai Chi Instructors

Tai chi is a series of slow, gentle movements designed to enhance mind and body function. It is usually practiced outdoors and is a moving meditation. Each move has a symbolic meaning. The Chinese practice tai chi every morning, and it is believed to be the most widely practiced exercise in the world. Because of its gentle nature, it is appropriate for any age. Research studies show the movements improve awareness of different body parts and have positive effects on the heart and blood vessels, the bones, the muscles, and even the nervous system. Its tranquil nature reduces stress and stress-related conditions. To find a tai chi teacher, go to http://lifematters.com/taieach.html.

Yoga Teachers

Yoga in Sanskrit means union of the different aspects of a person. *Hatha yoga* is a way of controlling the mind through mastery of the body, using postures and breathing conducive to meditation and bodily control. Yogic body postures make up the majority of hatha yoga, which has been found to help blood pressure, depression, and osteoporosis and to aid in menopausal discomfort. Each posture was inspired by the natural surroundings of ancient India and named for them—for example, the tree pose, the cobra pose, and so on. When the posture is pronounced, *asana* is added, which means calm, steady state, or seat. Asana also implies that each posture is a prelude to the ultimate goal of hatha yoga, being comfortable and healthy.

A qualified instructor is recommended, especially if health issues need to be addressed. Go to the American Yoga Association (http://www.americanyogaassociation.org) or to the International Association of Yoga Therapists (http://www.iayt.org).

■ Choosing a Practitioner

You probably spend a lot of time finding a good accountant, dentist, insurance company, babysitter, or auto mechanic. Make sure you use at least as much effort finding your health care practitioner. Prior to looking for a practitioner, decide on the qualities you want.

Gender

Consider whether you'd rather work with a male or female practitioner. Female physicians tend to spend more time with their patients than their male counterparts as validated by a study conducted at the University of California and published in the *Journal of the American Medical Women's Association*. The results provided evidence that female physicians spent a significantly greater proportion of visits on preventive services and counseling than male physicians, and male physicians devoted more time to technical practice behaviors and discussions of substance abuse.

A review of studies between 1967 and 2001 concluded that medical visits with female physicians averaged 2 minutes (10%) longer than those with male physicians. Female physicians engaged in significantly more communication that can be considered patient centered. They engaged in more active partnership behaviors, positive talk, psychosocial counseling, psychosocial question asking, and emotionally focused talk. Patients of female physicians spoke more overall, disclosed more biomedical and psychosocial information, and made more positive statements to their physicians than the patients of male physicians. Only male physicians in obstetrics and gynecology demonstrated higher levels of emotionally focused talk than their female colleagues.

Race

There hasn't been a lot of research on race and its effect on how you're treated, but one study showed that African American consumers who visit physicians of the same race rate their medical visits as more satisfying and participatory than those who see physicians of other races. Race-concordant visits are longer and characterized by more positive patient feelings. The association between race concordance and higher ratings of care is independent of patient-centered communication, suggesting that other factors, such as patient and physician attitudes, may be at work.

Another study examining referrals to specialists found that white physicians were more likely than black physicians to rate previous experience with the specialist and board certification to be of major importance. White physicians were somewhat less likely than black physicians to rate patient convenience to be of major importance.

Physician Practice Style

Style of physician–patient interaction has been shown to have an impact on health outcome. Researchers at Case Western Reserve University observed 2,881 patients visiting 138 family physicians for outpatient care in 84 community family practice offices in northeastern Ohio. Physicians with person-focused style rated highest on four of five measures of quality of the physician–patient relationship and patient satisfaction. Physicians with a high control style were lowest or next to lowest on outcomes. Physicians with a person-focused style granted the longest visits, while high-control physicians held the shortest visits—a difference of 2 minutes per visit on average. The differences were not explained away by patient and physician age and gender.

Physician Communication Style

Physician communication style is important to your health. Studies have shown when patients are informed and involved in decision making, they are more apt to follow medical recommendations and to carry out more health-related behavior changes. A major study reported in the *Journal of the American Board of Family Practice* provided a review of studies from 1975 to 2000 of office interactions between primary care physicians and patients that evaluated these interactions using neutral observers who coded what they saw or heard. The researchers concluded that physicians should focus on patient satisfaction, understanding, empathy, courtesy, friendliness, reassurance, support, and encouragement, answering questions, giving explanations, and reinforcing good feelings about patient actions. Physicians ought to listen, provide health education, summarize patient statements, talk on the patient's level, and clarify what they mean. Patient satisfaction after a visit was decreased by excessive biomedical question asking and interrupting patients when they were speaking. Physicians ought to avoid being unduly dominant, angry, nervous, and directive. Several researchers also emphasized the importance of patients being involved in decisions about their care.

A study conducted at the Johns Hopkins University School of Hygiene and Public Health examined communication patterns of primary care physicians. The researchers found five distinct communication patterns: (1) narrowly biomedical, characterized by closed-ended medical questions and biomedical talk that occurred in 32% of the visits; (2) expanded biomedical, like the restricted pattern but with moderate levels of psychosocial discussion occurring in 33% of the visits; (3) biopsychosocial, reflecting a balance of psychosocial and biomedical topics in 20% of the visits; (4) psychosocial, characterized by psychosocial exchange in 8% of the visits; and (5) consumerist, characterized primarily by patient questions and physician information giving in 8% of the visits. Biomedically focused visits were used more often with more sick, older, and lower-income patients by younger male physicians. Physician satisfaction was lowest in the narrowly biomedical pattern and highest in the consumerist pattern, while patient satisfaction was highest in the psychosocial pattern.

Referral to Specialists

Primary care physicians may refer you to a specialist. What do they consider to be important elements about the specialist to whom they're referring you? One study found the most important criteria were medical skill, appointment timeliness, insurance coverage, previous experience with the specialist, quality of specialist communication, specialist efforts to return the patient to the primary physician for care, and the likelihood of good patient–specialist rapport.

Similarity to Other Practitioners

A study of family physicians (FPs) and naturopathic practitioners (NPs) found that patients perceived no difference in patient-centered care between FPs and NPs. The same was true of nurse practitioners and physicians. In a study conducted at the University of Texas at Arlington, clinic patients perceived no difference in health and satisfaction with care whether the care was given by a nurse practitioner or a primary care physician.

Consumer Beliefs

Effective communication is a critical component of quality health care. A study at Texas A&M University examined the control exerted over the practitioner–consumer relationship by practitioners and consumers. Patients who preferred shared control were more active, expressing more opinions, concerns, and questions than consumers oriented toward physician control. Physicians used more partnership building with male patients. Approximately 14% of patient participation was prompted by physician partnership building, and 33% of physician partnership building was in response to active patient participation. If you ask more questions and express more opinions and concerns, you're more apt to evoke partnership building in your practitioner.

Cost/Coverage

Many holistic and complementary practitioners are not covered by health maintenance organizations (HMOs) or insurance plans. You may have to decide whether you're willing to pay additional money or a copayment to work with one.

Credentials

Many practitioners hang their credentials on their office wall, but you have a right to ask practitioners where they went to school and what specific things they learned in school or in continuing education courses that could make them especially helpful to you.

Experience/Success

In addition to education, practitioners' experience may be important to you. Feel free to ask how many menopausal women they've worked with and their success rate.

Certification

Being board certified means a practitioner has had clinical experience and passed a competency exam in a particular area. If this is important to you, ask practitioners you're considering whether they are board certified. Although board certification doesn't guarantee a practitioner can help you, it is one measure you can use to evaluate the competency of a practitioner.

Disciplinary Action

You may want to know if a practitioner has had any disciplinary actions taken against him or her. In some states you can find this information about physicians and nurse practitioners on the state's health department Web site. Do an Internet search using terms such as Department of Health, Florida (or whatever state you live in).

Flexible Hours

If you work or have other time constraints, a practitioner's office hours may be important. Call prior to making an appointment to find out hours of practice and if home visits are possible.

References

You may want to talk to other consumers who've used the practitioner's services. Ask for references, then call or e-mail them to ask whatever you'd like to know about the practitioner.

Screening Practitioner Candidates

Once you've decided the type(s) of practitioner(s) with whom you want to work, ask around. Friends, family, and other health care professionals can provide the names of practitioners they recommend. Ask for information about what they like and don't like about a practitioner and what their experiences have been with the health care provider.

When you've narrowed down your choices to a short list, start calling the practitioners. Speak with the office manager or the practitioner and ask the following questions. Add any others you have.

- Are you accepting new clients?
- Do I need a referral?
- What are your hours?
- Am I apt to get switched to another practitioner without advance notice?
- Who would I be likely to be switched to?
- How long am I apt to be kept waiting when I have an appointment?
- What fee do you charge per session?
- What insurance, Medicaid, and Medicare coverage do you accept?
- What copayments must I pay?
- What deductibles are due at my first visit?

- Is full payment required at the time of the appointment or can I work out a pay schedule?
- How long do I have to wait to get an appointment?
- Do you charge for missed appointments?
- How soon do you return phone calls?
- Do you give advice over the phone or by e-mail?
- Do you provide sessions at home or work?
- Do you provide handouts for treatment options and homework, and do you involve me in treatment decisions?
- Do you perform lab work in your own office or send it out to an independent laboratory?
- Can you provide references from consumers who have used your services?

If you can't get answers to these questions and any other information you require to make an informed decision, move on to another practitioner. Relationships with health care providers who refuse to respect your right to be involved in decisions about your care aren't in your best interest.

When you've eliminated most practitioners based on these questions, you may want to visit the practitioner's office and/or set up an appointment with the practitioner to learn more. Be aware that you may be charged for this visit. Many of the answers, and maybe most, can be answered by observing the practitioner and staff in action and examining the forms used in the practice. The information you gather will help you decide which one of the health care providers suits your needs best. Here are some other things to ask before settling on a practitioner:

- Can you give me samples of your diagnostic, evaluation, health education, and prevention forms?
- Who are the alternative/complementary practitioners you use for referrals?
- What side effects does this treatment have?

- Do you have any literature about this medication (treatment) I can have?
- Do I get to undress and dress in private?
- What treatment and payment options do I have?
- Are you interested in teaching me about the medicines or treatments you prescribe?
- What kind of input do I have into decisions about my care?
- How comfortable are you answering my questions about health care?
- How interested are you in my opinions and feelings?

Also observe: Do staff members . . .

- treat you with respect?
- gossip or share private information about other clients?

Does the practitioner . . .

- keep you waiting for your appointment?
- take time to learn about you, your background, and your lifestyle?
- patiently explain all treatments/medications and their pros and cons?
- answer all your questions to your satisfaction?
- admit or show through facial expression that he or she isn't comfortable answering your questions?
- act irritated or impatient or ignore your requests for explanations?
- talk about research findings you found in this book, in the media, or online?
- take written materials about you and research findings you bring in and promise to read them?
- dismiss all information but his or hers as quackery or uninformed?

When you return from your first visit, reevaluate your selection. If you're not comfortable, motivated, and feel you've been treated well, visit another practitioner on your list.

■ Communicating with Your Practitioner

You are the one most interested in staying well and the best person to keep track of all your health care records. Get a notebook with a divider. Ask for copies, not a handwritten summary, of all notes and tests (laboratory and otherwise) and provide a stamped self-addressed envelope so the office manager knows you're serious. Keep all information organized by date. Use dividers to separate the notebook by lab work, consultation, X-ray reports, and so on, for easy reference.

Keep track of dates of visits to practitioners, injections, vaccinations, special treatments, diagnostic procedures, dosage level of medication and when begun and ended, blood test results, diagnosed diseases, surgeries, hospitalizations, major emotional and physical stresses, and your own progress notes (menopause changes, how they affect your life, nutrition/stress management/herbal and other actions taken to reduce changes, which ones work and which ones don't).

■ Preparing for Appointments

Time is money for practitioners, so go to your health care appointments well organized and you're more likely to be treated with respect. To have a successful visit:

• Fax ahead or mail in advance any research articles or information you want your practitioner to read.

• Bring a friend or family member who is assertive and who can speak up for you in a diplomatic way. If your practitioner gives you a hard time about bringing someone along, hold your line. You're paying the bill and should be able to decide whom to bring into the examining and treatment room with you. As long as the person who accompanies you doesn't have an active communicable infection and refrains from touching anything in the room, there shouldn't be a problem. Even better, bring a health care professional with you. Be sure you share your agenda with your friend or provide a copy of your list so you both know the points you want to cover. That person can also take notes or help you re-create what happened after the appointment ends.

- Bring a copy of the names and dosages of all medications, supplements, and herbs you are taking as well as any other complementary treatment you're using.

- Treat each appointment as if it were an important business meeting, which it is. The business is your health, so take it seriously. Remember: the practitioner works for you. Dress for success by wearing a suit. Avoid apologizing for asking for information and explanations. You deserve to know the rationale behind any treatment or medication that is prescribed.

- Write down your main concerns and present them in the order of importance to you.

- Take notes on your practitioners' comments whenever you can. Between you and your friend, you should have all important points covered.

- Ask all your questions. Whenever the practitioner says something you don't understand, say, "I'm not sure I understand what you mean. Would you please repeat it in less technical language?"

Practitioner Checklist

As you gather information about practitioners, rate each item according to its importance to you, then compare practitioners, choosing the one(s) who most closely resembles your required qualities.

Practitioner Qualities	Important	Not Important
1. Is the same gender as I am		
2. Is the same race as I am		
3. Shares decision making with me		
4. Shows interest in my opinions and feelings		
5. Is supportive		
6. Is respectful		
7. Explains rationale for tests and treatments		
8. Explains how referral decisions are made		
9. Cost for treatment is covered by my insurance		
10. Credentials are adequate to provide good treatment		
11. Has had experience and success with similar clients		
12. Is board certified in a relevant specialty		
13. Has no disciplinary action in effect		
14. Has flexible hours of treatment		
15. Provides client references		
16. Is accepting new clients		
17. Will take me on without a referral		
18. Sees me within 5 minutes of my appointment time		
19. Requires copayment		

Practitioner Qualities	Important	Not Important
20. Allows me to work out a pay schedule	_____	_____
21. Never switches me to another practitioner without advanced notice	_____	_____
22. Fits me in for an appointment	_____	_____
23. Doesn't charge for missed appointments when notified within 24 hours	_____	_____
24. Returns my phone calls promptly	_____	_____
25. Is willing to give advice over the phone or by e-mail	_____	_____
26. Provides handouts about medication and treatment options and their side effects	_____	_____
27. Sends out blood and other lab tests to an independent lab	_____	_____
28. Refers to alternative/complementary practitioners	_____	_____
29. Staff is professional and does not gossip about or share information about other clients in my presence	_____	_____
30. Takes time to learn about me, my background and lifestyle	_____	_____
31. Patiently explains all treatments/medications and their pros and cons	_____	_____
33. Answers all my questions to my satisfaction	_____	_____
34. Takes whatever written materials about me or research findings I provide and discusses them with me	_____	_____

Remember that your primary health practitioner needs to be your partner in wellness decisions. Find a compassionate, informed person who will work with you, not dictate to you, so together you can find the right solutions for you.

Putting It All Together: Your Menopause Success Plan

For more than 15 years, I've been on a mission to learn all I can about menopause not only to help myself but to pass on what I've learned to you. Menopause is not a disease, so there is no cure, no silver bullet, and no perfect practitioner—except maybe you.

The only way menopause will work for you is if you use the information in this book to develop your own personalized wellness plan. If you invest the time and effort required to make a plan and follow it through, you will be way ahead of the game and well on your way to being well with menopause.

Each menopause journey is unique. The key is to find the right approach for you.

■ Attitude Is Important

Viewing menopause as a normal process is a start in the right direction. But it's not all roses, even when you find the right mix of self-care to help you feel energetic. While there may be a few things to cheer about, such as the fact you don't have to worry about becoming pregnant and you no longer have to deal with menstrual periods, there may be a few things to grieve.

> *Jetta, a 48-year-old grandmother, was able to end her bladder and vaginal discomfort and reduce the hot flashes that accompanied her menopause. Her husband, whom I'd seen for his diabetes a few years earlier, called me because he couldn't understand why his wife was so sad. He asked me if he should try to cheer her up, maybe take her on a vacation or a long weekend. I told him it wasn't unusual for women to feel a sense of loss about the way their body has changed. If you define yourself as a childbearer and mother, losing that ability can be sad. Jetta was able to talk with her husband about her feelings.*

Whether or not you feel sad about losing your ability to have children, try to remain positive about your menopause process. The more you invest yourself in dealing with the negative aspects of menopause, the more apt you are to have a positive experience.

■ Coordinate Your Wellness Team

Once you've chosen your wellness team, it will be up to you to coordinate their efforts. At least you've chosen them, so you know they'll be on your side and supportive of your objectives.

At certain times, you might have to be assertive, encouraging practitioners to talk to one another so your treatment is coordinated. You can help by . . .

- Giving each practitioner a current list of your drugs, nutritional supplements, herbs, and complementary and self-care measures

- Asking each practitioner to provide a summary of your work together and give you a copy
- Encouraging practitioners to speak with one another if there is any disagreement among them and including you in the discussion, perhaps via a conference call

If one or more of your practitioners refuses to collaborate, this is a red flag that it's time to replace them with more cooperative team members.

When you have a working team, be sure to put their names and specialties in your wellness plan notebook, along with their phone number, cell number, fax number, and other identifying information.

■ Choosing Your Self-Care Options

Anna, a 52-year-old accountant, came to me because she didn't want to take hormones and drugs and wanted a natural menopause. She'd been suffering through increased menstrual bleeding alternating with no period, hot flashes, dizziness, depression, and cold hands. Her mother had undergone a double mastectomy after being diagnosed with breast cancer, and Anna was afraid. Using the information in chapters 4 through 9, I coached Anna to develop her own menopause wellness plan. She agreed not to write down any action that she didn't think she would follow. That way, we built in more chances for success.

Check out Anna's plan. You'll notice that the possible changes run down the left side of the form and the types of approaches run across the top of the form. Anna filled in only the parts that related to her changes and only used the suggestions from chapters 4 through 9 that appealed to her. She wrote N/A for not applicable in the areas that didn't apply.

Anna's Living Well with Menopause Plan

Menopause Changes	Nutrition	Herbs	Environment	Exercise	Stress Reduction/ Healing	Relation-ships
Breast cancer and other cancers	Eat more apples, seeds, whole-grain cereals and breads, sardines, almonds, asparagus, broccoli, dandelion greens, watercress, chickory, oats, lima beans, soy products, sunflower seeds, onions, maitake mushrooms, berries. No alcohol or coffee. Take 1,500 mg calcium citrate daily in divided doses.	Drink red clover tea.	Use distilled water; avoid pesticides.	Female deer exercise.	Picture my breasts healthy and pink.	Tell Todd I don't want to end up like my mom, so please bear with menu changes. Besides, they might help him lose the weight he wants to lose.
Cold hands	Eat more peppers, parsley, alfalfa sprouts, sweet potatoes.	Take ginger and cayenne.	Use ginger compresses.	Finger pulls.	Picture warmth moving into my hands.	Ask Todd not to disturb me while I'm listening to my relaxation tape.
Depression, nervousness, and irritability	Eat more eggs, poultry, salmon, almonds, mackerel, peas, wheat germ, figs, carrots, corn, walnuts, avocados, bananas, cantaloupe, tempeh.	Drink ginseng tea; St. John's-wort.	Volunteer to read to nursing home residents.	Yoga class Tuesday and Friday.	Read *Feeling Good: The New Mood Therapy*.	Apologize to Todd for being so irritable and depressed. Ask for his cooperation with time-outs when I need them.
Dizziness	Eat more beets, lentils, millet, pears, pumpkin seeds, plantains.	Take gingko biloba 60 mg twice a day.	Stop playing virtual reality games on computer.	Cawthorne-Cooksey exercises.	Take qigong classes.	Play catch with Todd.
Fatigue	N/A					
Hair loss/ thinning	N/A					
Headaches	N/A					
Heart disease	N/A					

Anna's Living Well with Menopause Plan

Menopause Changes	Nutrition	Herbs	Environment	Exercise	Stress Reduction/ Healing	Relation-ships
Hot flashes	Stop eating sugary foods and drinking hot beverages. Drink soy milk and add flaxseed to cereal.	Take black cohosh 40 mg a day.	Use cooling mist and fans.	Walk every night after dinner.	Relaxing my body and picturing me cool and calm.	Ask Todd to help by not arguing.
Insomnia/ sleep problems	N/A					
Itchiness	N/A					
Joint and muscle pain	N/A					
Memory loss and fuzzy thinking	N/A					
Menstrual Bleeding	Stop eating red meat and dairy products. Eat more purple grapes, prunes, raisins, blackstrap molasses, kelp, garlic, alfalfa sprouts, wheat germ, raw spinach, cabbage, cauliflower, tomatoes.	Drink red raspberry tea; take turmeric capsules.	Take Stop Smoking class at Lung Association.	Garden.	Picture my periods slowly tapering off.	Tell Todd how much my heavy bleeding scares me; ask for his support.
Osteoporosis	N/A					
Sex drive reduction and intercourse discomfort	N/A					
Skin problems	N/A					
Urinary symptoms	N/A					
Weight gain	N/A					

Ginger, a 49-year-old mother of twins and a licensed social worker complained of different menopause changes than Anna, which is not unusual. Women rarely suffer from all possible menopause changes. Ginger's complaints were fatigue, losing hair, headaches, fear of dying from the heart condition that had taken her father in his 50s, insomnia, low sex drive, urine leakage, and weight gain. Using information found in chapters 4 through 9, I helped her construct her Living Well with Menopause Plan.

Ginger's Living Well with Menopause Plan

Menopause Changes	Nutrition	Herbs	Environment	Exercise	Stress Reduction/ Healing	Relation- ships
Breast cancer and other cancers		N/A				
Cold hands		N/A				
Depression, nervousness, and irritability		N/A				
Dizziness		N/A				
Fatigue	Eat more salmon, dates, green leafy vegetables, almonds, tofu, brown rice, split peas, onions, strawberries, cauliflower, blackstrap molasses, alfalfa sprouts.	Take 1–2 grams ginseng daily.	Take a time management course.	Dance, walk, or cycle each day; use shiatsu to invigorate.	Practice getting my body relaxed with a relaxation tape and picturing myself energetic and strong.	Tell my partner about my fatigue. Ask for help with house-hold tasks.
Hair loss/ thinning	No caffeine. Eat more whole-grain bread and cereals, plums, raisins, broccoli, dandelion greens, bananas, tempeh, avocados. Cook in iron pots. Take coenzyme Q10.	Drink horse-tail tea and oatstraw tea.	Avoid hair dryers. Don't comb hair when it's wet and never brush.	Massage my scalp daily and tug my hair.	Picture circulation increasing to my scalp.	Tell my partner about my hair loss and that I'll be eating foods and taking herbs to help.

Ginger's Living Well with Menopause Plan

Menopause Changes	Nutrition	Herbs	Environment	Exercise	Stress Reduction/ Healing	Relation- ships
Headaches	No caffeine, lunch meat, cheese, beer, wine, MSG, artificial sweeteners, roasted nuts, chocolate, citrus juices, pickled cabbage. Eat low-fat foods, spinach, lima beans, sunflower seeds.	Take black cohosh (follow directions on the label).	Avoid plastics. Replace with natural materials.	Use acupressure daily and massage webbing between thumb and index finger.	Do yoga: child pose and neck roll.	Teach my partner about guided imagery for pain.
Heart disease	Eat almonds, apples, grapes, filberts, prunes, sesame seeds, turnip greens, watercress, yellow squash, papaya, beets, flaxseeds, figs, maitake mushrooms, radishes, Swiss chard.	Take red clover 50 mg/day.	Spend 10 minutes in the sun three times a week. Stay away from smoke.	Do complete arm massage.	Picture myself relaxing; take a qigong class.	Ask my partner to take a walk with with me after dinner every night.
Hot flashes	N/A					
Insomnia/ sleep problems	No caffeine or alcohol. Eat more brewer's nutritional yeast, carob, lentils, collards, fennel, wheat germ, oranges, cucumber, peanuts.	Drink chamomile tea at bedtime.	Avoid eating when unable to sleep. Keep a sleep log to identify what's keeping me awake. Take a lavender bath.	Do complex flexibility exercises prior to sleep.	Listen to my relaxation tape; change my negative thoughts about sleep.	Ask my partner to massage my feet.
Itchiness	N/A					
Joint and muscle pain	N/A					
Memory loss and fuzzy thinking	N/A					
Menstrual bleeding		N/A				

Ginger's Living Well with Menopause Plan

Menopause Changes	Nutrition	Herbs	Environment	Exercise	Stress Reduction/ Healing	Relation- ships
Osteoporosis	N/A					
Sex drive reduction and intercourse discomfort	Eat more soy cheese, tempeh, tofu, whole-grain oat cereal and bread.	Take one or two damiana capsules, 400 mg, prior to lovemaking.	Stop using douches. Use aphrodisiac scents in bedroom. Give each other a massage prior lovemaking.	Do 12 abdominal contractions every day.	Devise a sexual intercourse hierarchy and practice it until I'm relaxed and calm.	Thank my partner for his patience and and suggest we both take damiana before sex.
Skin problems	N/A					
Urinary symptoms	Avoid spices, tomatoes, citrus juice, and fruit. Eat more blueberries, basil, coriander, oregano, fresh pineapple, cabbage, brussels sprouts, eggs, watermelon.	Drink 1 or 2 cups nettle tea a day.	Avoid aluminum cookware. Buy reverse osmosis water filter or drink and cook with distilled water.	Do 100 Kegels every day.	Use self-hypnosis suggestions: My bladder is toned and strengthening. I am in charge of my urination.	Thank my partner for stopping at rest rooms so often.
Weight gain	Avoid meat and dairy products. Drink 8–10 glasses of water a day. Eat 4–6 small meals a day but never after 7 p.m. Eat lots of organic fruits and vegetables.	Take licorice, 3.5 grams a day for 2 months.	Throw out or give away all trans-fats, sugar and sugary foods, and food additives. Stock up on organic fruits, vegetables, soy foods, and whole-grain breads and cereals.	Do alternate leg raises, standing side bend, and the crane.	Have two sessions with a hynotherapist or purchase a weight-loss self-hypnosis tape.	Thank my partner for reminding me not to eat too much and for not bringing home pizza or ice cream.

The blank form for your wellness plan appears below. Copy it for your own use. (A downloadable version of this form is also available online at http://Menopause.bellaonline.com.)

Your Living Well with Menopause Plan

Menopause Changes	Nutrition	Herbs	Environment	Exercise	Stress Reduction/ Healing	Relation- ships
Breast cancer and other cancers						
Cold hands						
Depression, nervousness, and irritability						
Dizziness						
Fatigue						
Hair loss/ thinning						
Headaches						
Heart disease						
Hot flashes						
Insomnia/ sleep problems						

Your Living Well with Menopause Plan

Menopause Changes	Nutrition	Herbs	Environment	Exercise	Stress Reduction/ Healing	Relation- ships
Itchiness						
Joint and muscle pain						
Memory loss and fuzzy thinking						
Menstrual bleeding						
Osteoporosis						
Sex drive reduction and intercourse discomfort						
Skin problems						
Urinary symptoms						
Weight gain						

I hope the information, ideas, and resources in this book will inspire you and guide you toward finding your optimal wellness team and creating your own menopause wellness plan. Write to me about your experiences, questions, ideas, and comments on the book, or if you want to share your own menopause story. You can contact me by e-mail or sign up for my Menopause Newsletter at http://meno pause.bellaonline.com.

Best wishes on your menopause journey. May it be the best time of your life!

Appendix

RESOURCES

I've assembled a list of useful resources to help you find the information and support you need before, during, and after menopause. Resources, by their nature, are subject to change. If you come across out-of-date information, go to my Web site at http://menopause.bellaonline.com for updates. You can e-mail me from there, join a forum, and talk to your menopausal peers or sign up for *Menopause at Bellaonline,* my newsletter, which tells you about the latest articles and information available on the topic.

If you don't have Web site or e-mail access at home, work, or your local library, please contact me by writing to HarperCollins Publishers, 10 East 53rd Street, New York, NY 10022-5299.

■ Menopause Forum

You can find Menopause Forum on my Menopause Web site by clicking on Boards or Forums at the top or bottom of any article page at http://menopause.bellaonline.com. Talk to women just like you who are struggling with similar issues. I go there, too, and provide information.

■ Menopause Newsletter

Menopause at Bellaonline is my free newsletter designed to keep women in perimenopause up-to-date on the latest information, both conventional and alternative/complementary, to enhance their ability to live well. I scour the medical journals and alternative/holistic/complementary sources in the United States and around the world looking for information to help you have a more pleasant menopause experience. Sign up at http://menopause.bellaonline.com.

■ Other Menopause-Related Web Sites and Toll-Free Phone Numbers

Acupuncture

For information on acupuncture and its use with menopause changes or practitioners in your geographical area, go to the following Web sites:

American Academy of Medical Acupuncture
Internet Address: http://www.medicalacupuncture.org

American Association of Oriental Medicine
Internet Address: http://www.aaom.org

Aging Issues

Worried about aging? Go to the Web sites below for ideas and information.

National Institute on Aging
Internet Address: http://www.nih.gov/nia
Toll-Free: (800) 222-2225; (800) 222-4225 (TTY)

Older Women's League (OWL)
Internet Address: http://www.owl-national.org
E-mail: owlinfo@owl-national.org
Toll-Free: (800) 825-3695

Alternative/Complementary/Holistic Issues and Practitioners

Want to learn about self-care, alternative, complementary and/or holistic approaches to menopause or to find practitioners in your geographical area, go to the Web sites below.

American Holistic Health Association
Internet Address: http://www.ahha.org

American Holistic Medical Association
Internet Address: http://www.holisticmedicine.org

American Holistic Nurses' Association
Internet Address: http://www.ahna.org
Toll-Free: (800) 278-2462

Dr. Andrew Weil's Practitioner Database
Internet Address: http://www.drweil.com

Holistic Health at Bellaonline.com
Provides a weekly e-newsletter, a forum for discussion of self-care, and more than 100 articles.
Internet Address: http://HolisticHealth.bellaonline.com

Menopause at Bellaonline.com
Provides more than 100 menopause articles, a free weekly newsletter, and a forum for discussion.
Internet Address: http://Menopause.bellaonline.com

National Center for Complementary and Alternative Medicine
Provides a free newsletter and information about ongoing research and research centers.
Internet Address: http://www.nccam.nih.gov
Publication: http://nccam.nih.gov.health/alerts/menopause

Cancer

Are you at high risk for cancer? Many women are after menopause. Check in with the Web site below for more information.

National Cancer Institute
Internet Address: http://cis.nci.nih.gov
Toll-Free: (800) 332-8615

Communication/Couples Relationships

Communication and sexual relationships can change radically during perimenopause. See this Web site for available information.

Virginia Johnson Masters Learning Center
Internet Address: http://www.vjmlc.com
Toll-Free: (888) 937-3528

Food and Drug Issues

Worried about the effects of the prescription or over-the-counter drugs on your menopause changes? Check in with this Web site.

Food and Drug Administration (FDA)
Office on Women's Health
Internet Address: http://www.fda.gov/womens/menopause

Guided Imagery

Guided imagery can be an effective approach for many menopause changes. Check the following Web site for practitioners and approaches.

Academy for Guided Imagery
Internet Address: http://www.academyforguidedimagery.com

Health/Medical News Web Sites

Want health and medical news Web sites? The *New York Times* and/or Reuters can help supply you with up-to-date information.

New York Times
Internet Address: http://www.nytimes.com
(Go to the Women's Health section.)
or http://yourhealthdaily.com

Reuter's Health
Internet Address: http://www.reutershealth.com

Herbs

Herbs can be helpful for some menopause changes. Check the following Web site for information on herbs and practitioners.

American Herbalists Guild
Internet Address: http://www.americanherbalistsguild.com

Hypnosis

Hypnosis can provide help with stress, anxiety, depression, as well as physical changes. For practitioners and information on hypnosis, visit the following Web site.

American Society of Clinical Hypnosis
Internet Address: http://www.asch.net

Hysterectomy

Contact one or more of the groups below for information to help you make a decision about having a hysterectomy, medical guidelines for appropriate hysterectomies, and what to do before and after a hysterectomy.

Agency for Healthcare Research and Quality
Internet Address: http://www.ahcpr.gov

American College of Obstetricians and Gynecologists
Internet Address: http://www.acog.com
Toll-Free: (800) 762-2264

Association of Women's Health, Obstetric, and Neonatal Nurses
Internet Address: http://www.awhonn.org

Menopause at Bellaonline.com
Internet Address: http://Menopause.bellaonline.com

National Women's Health Information Center
Internet Address: http://www.4woman.org
Toll-Free: (800) 994-9662

National Women's Health Resource Center
Internet Address: http://www.healthywomen.org

Massage
For information on how massage may benefit you and to find a practitioner in your geographical area, click on the following Web sites.

American Massage Therapy Association
Internet Address: http://www.amtamassage.org

Association of Bodywork and Massage Professionals
Internet Address: http://www.healthydoctors.com

National Association of Nurse Massage Therapists
Internet Address: http://www.nanmt.org
Toll-Free: (800) 262-4017

Medical Research Web Sites

Search the following Web sites for research abstracts on menopause topics. Begin with the National Library of Medicine, where you can find abstracts of current and past research that you can print out and share with your health care practitioner.

National Library of Medicine Searchable Database
Internet Address: http://www.pubmed.com

Medscape
Internet Address: http://www.medscape.com

Journal of the American Medical Association (JAMA)
Internet Address: http://www.ama-assn.org

New England Journal of Medicine
Internet Address: http://www.nejm.org

British Medical Journal
Internet Address: http://www.bmj.com

Menopause

Depending on your needs, choose from the Web sites below.

Menopause at Bellaonline.com
Menopause articles and a free newsletter that provides information about new articles available online. Uses a self-care, holistic approach and a visitor's forum where you can discuss menopause issues with peers who are going through (or have gone through) similar situations. Internet Address: http://menopause.bellaonline.com.

National Women's Health Network

Contact others interested in menopause issues.
Internet Address: http://www.nwhn.org

National Women's Health Resource Center

Menopause information of various kinds.
Internet Address: http://www.healthywomen.org
Toll-Free: (888) 406-9472

Women to Women

A private practice of physicians and nurse practitioners who offer a holistic and self-care approach to menopause.
Internet Address: http://www.womentowomen.com
Toll-Free: (800) 832-2342

North American Menopause Society

A more conventional approach to menopause.
Internet Address: http://www.menopause.org

Naturopaths

Of interest if you wish to take a drug-free approach to menopause and/or want to find a naturopath practitioner.

Natural Health Practitioners

Internet Address: http://www.nchm.net

Naturopathic Medicine Network

Internet Address: http://www.pandamedicine.com

Nutrition

Nutrition is a basic tool of self-care for menopause changes. The ADA does research on nutrition and its effect on your body.

American Dietetic Association (ADA)
Internet Address: http://www.eatright.org

Oriental Medicine

Oriental medicine has been around for thousands of years and many alternative and self-care approaches have been perfected. Visit the following site for more information and/or to find an Oriental medicine practitioner.

American Association of Oriental Medicine
Internet Address: http://www.aaom.org

Osteopathy

Osteopathy combines conventional medical practices of medicine and surgery with body manipulation procedures. If this appeals to you, visit the site that follows for information and to find a practitioner.

American Academy of Osteopathy
Internet Address: http://www.academyofosteopathy.org

Osteoporosis

Osteoporosis risk increases after menopause. For more information, go to the Web site below.

National Osteoporosis Foundation
Internet Address: http://www.nof.org

Reflexology

Reflexology is a method of massaging the foot, which thereby affects the rest of the body. For more information or to find a practitioner, contact the Web site below.

Reflexology Organizations
Internet Address: http://www.reflexology.org

Relaxation Therapy

Are you uptight? Nervous? Relaxation therapy may be perfect for you. For more information and/or to find a therapist, visit the Web site below.

Relaxation Therapists
Internet Address: http://www.nchm.net/DANHP/relax.htm

Sexual Relationships

Menopause changes can affect your sexual relationship. For more information go to the Web site or call the toll-free number below.

Virginia Johnson Masters Learning Center
Internet Address: http://www.vjmlc.com
Toll-Free: (888) 937-3528

Smoking Cessation

Do you want to quit smoking, but haven't been able to? Visit the Web sites below for information on how to quit and how to get support for quitting. Your local lung association may also offer free workshops on smoking cessation. Find it in your local phone book.
Internet Address: http://www.lungusa.org/tobacco
Internet Address: http://www.ashline.org
Internet Address: http://www.cancer.ca (Search for "tobacco.")
Internet Address: http://www.stop.tabac.ch

Tai Chi

Tai Chi is a form of movement that can help heal body, mind, and spirit. For more information or to find workshops or studios near you, go to the Web site below.

Tai Chi Workshops
Internet Address: http://www.lifematters.com

Yoga

American Yoga Association
Internet Address: http://www.americanyogaassociation.org

Association of Yoga Therapists
Internet Address: http://www.iayt.org

■ Menopause-Related Books

De-Stress, Weigh Less: A Six-Step No-Diet Plan for Relaxing Your Way to Permanent Weight Loss
P. J. Rosch, MD, and C. C. Clark, ARNP
　Weight gain is common after menopause. If you're on a weight loss–weight gain cycle, this book may help you. It focuses on the stress that leads to binge eating and provides menus, ways to train yourself so you don't overeat, exercise ideas, suggestions for subduing other life stressors, and tips on keeping the weight off for good.

Menopausal Years—The Wise Woman Way
S. S. Weed
　This book has been the bible for many perimenopausal women. Susan Weed provides information about using herbs safely for ages 30 to 90.

Women's Bodies, Women's Wisdom: Creating Physical and Emotional Health and Healing
C. Northrup, MD
　The strength of this book is its focus on the effect of emotions on the body, how "naming" your experience can dramatically improve

your health, and how to enhance your positive energy flow to improve your well-being.

A Woman's Best Medicine: Health, Happiness and Long Life Through Ayur-Veda

N. Lonsdorf, MD, V. Butler, MD, and M. Brown, PhD

This book provides in-depth information about how to use the time-tested Ayur-Vedic program to help develop and use your self-knowledge to deal with the high-stress demands of contemporary life.

Natural Women's Health: A Guide to Healthy Living for Women of Any Age

L. Wharton, Registered Acupuncturist and Naturopath

Lynda Wharton believes the healthiest decision any woman can make is to choose to take control of her own health care. Her book provides the specifics for doing just that, and it gives invaluable information for coping with and recovering from yeast infections, anemia, cystitis, fibroids, genital herpes, and osteoporosis.

American Holistic Nurses' Association Guide to Common Chronic Conditions: Self-Care Options to Complement Your Doctor's Advice

C. C. Clark

This book discusses conventional and self-care approaches for conditions that often plague women during perimenopause. Nearly all are based on solid research. Topics that relate to menopause include arthritis, cancer, carpal tunnel syndrome, chronic fatigue, depression, diabetes, digestive prolems, fibromyalgia, heart and blood vessel disorders, osteoporosis, overweight, pain, and sleep problems.

Prescription for Nutritional Healing

J. F. Balch, MD, and Phyllis A. Balch, CNC

Written by a certified nutritional counselor and a physician, this self-help approach to good health includes drug-free remedies using vitamins, minerals, herbs, and food supplements by various conditions. A great reference to have on hand. You'll refer to it often.

8 Weeks to Optimum Health

A. Weil, MD

Dr. Weil's book provides an 8-week, step-by-step guide to building up and nourishing your mind, body, and spirit, helping restore energy and resilience to your immune system. The suggestions are doable and effective. For an excellent vitamin advisor, go to Dr. Weil's Web site at http://www.drweil.com.

Prescription Alternatives: Hundreds of Safe, Natural, Prescription-Free Remedies to Restore Your Health & Energy

E. Mindell and V. Hopkins

Are you taking prescription or over-the-counter drugs that may be adding to your menopause woes? Get this book and find out. A great reference to have on hand.

The Stop Smoking Workbook: Your Guide to Healthy Quitting

L. Rust and A. Maximin

This handy workbook includes information on preparation for quitting (myths and facts about smoking, laying the foundation for successful quitting, and smoking as a habit), alternative coping techniques and strategies, the actual quitting process, establishing a healthy lifestyle, and maintaining a smoke-free environment.

REFERENCES

Chapter 1: Introduction

"Antidepressant-related deaths." *Clinical Psychiatry News,* 32(2): 41; 2004.

Buchanan, M. C., Villagran, M. M., and Ragan, S. L. "Women, menopause, and (Ms.) information: communication about the climacteric." *Health Communications* 14(1):99–119; 2002.

Korzy, M., and Wells, R. "HRT a big mistake, says health body." *The Age,* March 5, 2004. http://www.theage.com.au/articles/ 2004/03/05/10/1078464638331.html.

Lonsdorf, N., Butler, V., and Brown, M. *A Woman's Best Medicine.* New York: Jeremy P. Tarcher/Putnam, 1993.

"Menopause facts elude female doctors." *Washington Post,* September 9, 1998.

Rosch, P. "Whom does the FDA really protect?" *Health and Stress, the Newsletter of the American Institute of Stress,* no. 5, p. 2; 2004.

Chapter 2: Menopause: A Natural Process

"Bad sex: Not a laughing matter." *Hippocrates,* July 1999, p. 8.

"Chemotherapy for breast cancer appears to have subtle impact on memory, language." *Clinical Psychiatry News,* February 2004.

Clinical News: Women's Health "Life after hysterectomy: A positive view." *American Journal of Nursing,* January 1998, p. 10.

"Depression and cardiovascular sequelae in postmenopausal women: the Women's Health Institute (WHI)." *Archives of Internal Medicine* 164(3); 2004. http://ncbi.nlm.nih.gov.

Goodman, M. "Menopausal symptoms in cancer." http://www. cancersourcern.com/Nursing/CE/CECourse.cfm?couseid= 1366contentid=22577.

Grayson, C. E. "Your guide to menopause." WebMD, 2002. http://content.health.msn.com/content/article9/2953_504?

"Insomnia." *Women's Health Advocate.* November 1998, p. 3.

Love, S. "Myths of menopause." SusanLoveMD.org. Accessed December 2003 at http://www.susanlovemd.com/decision/h_2. htm.

Mastrangelo, R., and Gerchufsky, M. "Headache." *Advance for Nurse Practitioners,* December 1994, pp. 9–11.

Mayo, P. E. *The Healing Sorrow Workbook.* New Harbinger Publications, Inc., 2001.

Meyer, D. M., Powell, L. H., Wilson, R. S., Everson-Rose, S. A., Kravitz, H. M., et al. "A population based longitudinal study of cognitive functioning in the menopausal transition." *Neurology,* September 2000, pp. E9–10.

Northrup, C. "Menopause." *Complementary and Alternative Therapies in Primary Care* 24(4):921–946; 1998.

Northrup, C. *Women's Bodies, Women's Wisdom.* New York: Bantam Books, 1994.

Pavlovich-Danis, S. J. "Antidepressant warnings issued." *Nursing Spectrum,* June 1, 2004, FL, p. 17.

Pavlovich-Danis, S. J. "When can do fades to why bother: understanding depression in women." *Nursing Spectrum,* June 1, 2004, pp. 12–13, 20.

"Perimenopause." *Women's Health Advocate Newsletter* 5(8):1–8; 1998.

Prior, J. C. "Spinal bone loss and ovulatory disturbances." *New England Journal of Medicine* 323: 1221–1227; 1990.

Staropoli, C. A., Flaws, J. A., Bush, T. L., and Moulton, A. W. "Predictors of menopausal hot flashes." *Journal of Women's Health,* November 1998.

Sullivan, M. G. "Antidepressants, sex dysfunction may be linked." *Clinical Psychiatry News,* November 2003, p. 62.

Sullivan, M. G. "90 million Americans lack full health literacy." *Clinical Psychiatry News,* May 2004, p. 106.

Wassertheil-Smoller S., Shumaker, S., Ockene, J., et al. "Depression and cardiovascular sequelae in postmenopausal women: the Women's Health Initiative (WHI)." *Archives of Internal Medicine* 164:289–298; 2004.

Chapter 3: Medical Treatment

Ascherio, A., Chen, H., Schwarzschild, M. A., Zhang, S. M., Colditz, G. A., and Speizer, F. E. "Caffeine, postmenopausal estrogen, and risk of Parkinson's disease." *Neurology,* March 11, 2003, pp. 790–795.

Altman, L. K. "New study links hormones to breast cancer risk." *New York Times,* August 8, 2003.

Barr, R. G., Wentowski, C. C., Grodstein, F., Somers, S. C., Stampfer, M. J., et al. "Prospective study of postmenopausal hormone use and newly diagnosed asthma and chronic obstructive pulmonary disease." *Archives of Internal Medicine,* February 23, 2004, pp. 379–386.

Barrett-Connor, E., Wehren, L. E., Siris, E. S., Miller, P., Chen, Y. T., et al. "Recency and duration of postmenopausal hormone therapy: effects on bone mineral density and fracture risk in the National Osteoporosis Risk Assessment (NORA) study." *Menopause,* 10(5) September–October 2003, pp. 412–419.

Bernstein, S. J. Unnecessary hysterectomy. *Journal of the American Medical Association,* May 1993.

Boschert, S. "MDs no longer control health information." *Clinical Psychiatry News,* February 2004.

Broder, M. S. "Hysterectomies recommended prematurely." *Obsterics and Gynecology* 95(2):199–205; 2000.

Burki, R. "Menopause management, part 1: perimenopausal transition and early menopause." *The Clinical Advisor,* February 2002, pp. 38–47.

Chen, W. Y., Colditz, G. A., Rosner, B., Hankinson, S. E., Hunter, D. J., et al. "Use of postmenopausal hormones, alcohol, and risk for invasive breast cancer." *Annals of Internal Medicine,* November 19, 2002, pp. 798–804.

Cooley, H. M., Stankovich, J., and Jones, G. "The association between hormonal and reproductive factors and hand osteoarthritis." *Maturitas,* August 20, 2003, pp. 257–265.

DeMarco, C. "How to save your uterus." *Natural Solutions,* Fall 1994.

Frieden, J. "Clinical trials: The new frontier in fraud." *Clinical Psychiatry News,* February 2004.

Garrison, R., and Somer, E. "Trace minerals." *The Nutrition Desk Reference.* New Canaan, CT: Keats, 1995, pp. 182–237.

Goodman, M. "Menopausal symptoms in cancer." http://www.cancersourcern.com/Nursing/CE/CECourse.cfm?courseid=1366 contentid=22577.

Grayson, C. E. "Your guide to menopause." WebMD, 2003. http://content.health/msn.com/content/article/9/2953_504?

Hodis, H. N., Mack, W. J., Azen, S. P., Lobo, R. A., Shoupe, D., et al. "Hormone therapy and the progression of coronary-artery atherosclerosis in postmenopausal women." *New England Journal of Medicine,* August 7, 2003, pp. 535–545.

Hoibraaten, E., Qvigstad, E., Arnesen, H., Larsen, S., Wickstome, E., and Sandset, P. M. "Increased risk of recurrent venous thromboembolism during hormone replacement therapy—results of the randomized, double-blind, placebo-controlled estrogen in venous thromboembolism trial (EVTET)." *Thrombosis and Haemostasis,* December 2000, pp. 961–967.

Holmberg, L., and Anderson, H. "Breast cancer risk halts another HRT trial." *The Lancet* 363: 453–455; 2004.

Key, T. J., Appleby, P. N., Reeves, G. K., Roddam, A., Dorgan, J. F., et al. "Body mass index, serum sex hormones, and breast cancer risk in postmenopausal women." *Journal of the National Cancer Institute,* August 20, 2003, pp. 1218–1236.

Li, C. I., Malone, K. E., Porter, P. L., Weiss, N. S., Tang, M. T., et al. "Reproductive and anthropometric factors in relation to the risk of lobular and ductal breast carcinoma among women 65–79 years of age. *International Journal of Cancer,* November 20, 2003, pp. 647–651.

Lokkegaard, E., Pedersen, A. T., Heitmann, B. L., Jovanovic, Z., Keiding, N., et al. "Relation between hormone replacement therapy and ischaemic heart disease in women: prospective observational study." *British Medical Journal,* February 22, 2003, p. 426.

Mann, D. "Soy products, ginseng may lower breast cancer risk." *Medical Tribune,* November 27, 1997, p. 33.

Manson, J. E., Hsia, J., Johnson, K. C., Rossouw, J. E., Assaf, A. R., et al. "Estrogen plus progestin and the risk of coronary heart disease. *New England Journal of Medicine* August 7, 2003, pp. 523–534.

"Menopause." Prepared by the National Institute on Aging, Washington, D.C., February 29, 2004. http://openseason.com/annex/library/cic/X0058_menopaus.txt.hbig.

Murphy, J.L. *Nurse Practitioners' Prescribing Reference*. New York: Prescribing Reference, Inc., 2004.

National Women's Health Information Center. "Menopause." U.S. Department of Health and Human Services, Office on Women's Health. Accessed February 29, 2004. http://www.4woman.gov /faq/menopaus.htm.

Peters, S. "Menopause: A new era." *Advance for Nurse Practitioners*, July 1998, pp. 61–64.

Sievert, L.L. "The medicalization of female fertility—points of significance for the study of menopause." *Collegium Antropologicum*, June 2003, pp. 67–78.

Smith, S. "Hormone therapy's rise and fall: science lost its way, and women lost out." *Boston Globe*, July 20, 2003.

Sornay-Rendu, E., Garnero, P., Munoz, F., Duboeuf, F., and Delmas, P.D. "Effect of withdrawal of hormone replacement therapy on bone mass and bone turnover: the OFELY study. *Bone*, July 2003, pp. 159–66.

Uhler, M.L., Marks, J.W., and Judd, H.I. "Estrogen replacement therapy and gallbladder disease in postmenopausal women. *Menopause*, May–June 2000, pp. 162–167.

Wang, S.Y., and Lin, H.S. "Compost as a soil supplement increases the level of antioxidant compounds and oxygen radical absorbance capacity in strawberries." *Journal of Agricultural and Food Chemistry*, November 5, 2003, pp. 6844–6850.

Whitehead, M. "Treatments for menopausal and post-menopausal problems: present and future." *Bailliers Clinical Obstetrics and Gynecology*, September 10, 1996, pp. 515–530.

Chapter 4: Nutrition

Aanthke, F., Gotz, M., and Jarisch, R. "Histamine-free diet: treatment of choice for histamine-induced food intolerance and supporting treatment for chronic headaches." *Clinical and Experimental Allergy*, December 1993, pp. 982–985.

Abbott, R. D., Ando, F., Masaki, K. H., et al. "Dietary magnesium intake and the future risk of coronary heart disease (the Honolulu Heart Program)." *American Journal of Cardiology*, September 15, 2003, pp. 665–669.

Albertazzi, P., Pansini, F., Bonaccorsi, G., et al. "The effect of dietary soy supplementation on hot flashes." *Obstetrics and Gynecology*, 91: 6–11; 1998.

Arnett, T. "Regulation of bone cell function by acid-base balance." *Proceedings of the Nutrition Society*, May 2003, pp. 511–520.

Arts, I. C., Jacobs, D. R., Jr., Harnack, L. J., Gross, M., and Folson A. R. "Dietary catechins in relation to coronary heart disease death among postmenopausal women." *Epidemiology*, November 2001, pp. 668–675.

Barton, D. L., Loprinzi, C. L., Quella, S. K., Sloan, J. A., Veeder, M. H., et al. "Prospective evaluation of vitamin E for hot flashes in breast cancer survivors." *Journal of Clinical Oncology*, 15: 495–500; 1998.

Bell, K. M., Pion, L., Bunney, W. E., et al. "S-adenosylmethionine treatment of depression: a controlled trial." *American Journal of Psychiatry* 145:1110–1014; 1988.

Bic, Z., Blix, G. G., Hopp, H. P., Leslie, F. M., and Schell, M. J. "The influence of a low-fat diet on incidence and severity of migraine headaches." *Journal of Women's Health Gender Based Medicine*, June 1999, pp. 623–630.

Braam, L. A., Hoeks, A. P., Brouns, F., Hamulyak, K., Gerichhausen, M. J., and Vermeer, C. "Beneficial effects of vitamins D and K on the elastic properties of the vessel wall in postmenopausal women: a follow-up study." *Thrombosis and Haemostasis*, February 2004, pp. 373–380.

"Calcium: Mega-Nutrient, Maxi-Deficient. *The Energy Times* July/August 1999, p. 14.

Cassidy, A., Bingham, S., and Setchell, K.D. "Biological effects of a diet of soy protein rich in isoflavones on the menstrual cycle of premenopausal women. *American Journal of Clinical Nutrition* 60:333–340; 1994.

Casto, B.C., Kresty, L.A., Kraly, C.L., Pearl, D.K., Knoblock, T.J., et al. "Chemoprevention of oral cancer by black raspberries." *Anticancer Research*, November–December 2002, pp. 4005–4015.

Chiaffarino, F., Parazzini, F., La Vecchia, C., Chatenoud, L., Di Cintio, E., and Marsico, S. "Diet and uterine myomas." *Obstetrics and Gynecology* 94(3):395–398; 1999.

Chiechi, L.M., Putignano, G., Guerra, V., Schiavelli, M.P., Cisternino, A.M., and Carriero, C. "The effect of a soy rich diet on the vaginal epithelium in postmenopause: a randomized double blind trial." *Maturitas*, August 2003, pp. 241–246.

Chiu, H.F., Chang, C.C., and Yang, C.Y. "Magnesium and calcium in drinking water and risk of death from ovarian cancer." *Magnesium Research* 17(1):28–34; 2004.

Clark, C.D., Bassett, B., and Burge, M.R. "Effects of kelp supplementation on thyroid function in euthyroid subjects." *Endocrine Practice* 9(5):363–369; 2003.

Convit, A., Wolf, O.T., Tarshish, C., and de Leon, M.J. "Reduced glucose tolerance is associated with poor memory performance and hippocampal atrophy among normal adults." *Proceedings of the American Academy of Sciences* 100(4): 2014–22; 2003.

Cotter, A., and Cashman, K.D. "Genistein appears to prevent early postmenopausal bone loss as effectively as hormone replacement therapy." *Nutrition Reviews*, October 2003, pp. 346–351.

De Leo, V., Lanzetta, D., Cazzavacca, R., and Morgante, G. "Treatment of neurovegetative menopausal symptoms with a phytotherapeutic agent." *Minerva Ginecologica*, May 1998, pp. 207–211.

Ding, M., Lu, Y., Bowman, L., Huang, C., Leonard, S., Wang, L., Vallyathan, V., Castranova, V., and Shi, X. "Inhibition of AP-1 and neoplastic transformation by fresh apple peel extract."

Journal of Biology and Chemistry, March 12, 2004, pp. 10, 670–110, 676.

Duffy, R., Wiseman, H., and File, S. E. "Improved cognitive function in postmenopausal women after 12 weeks of consumption of a soy extract containing isoflavones." *Pharmacology and Biochemical Behavior* 75(3):721–729; 2003.

Elgayyar, M., Draughon, F. A., Golden, D. A., and Mount, J. R. "Antimicrobial activity of essential oils from plants against selected pathogenic and saprophytic microorganisms." *Journal of Food Protection,* July 2001, pp. 1019–1024.

Fairfield, K. M., Hunter, D. J., Colditz, G. A., Fuchs, C. S., Cramer, D. W., et al. "A prospective study of dietary lactose and ovarian cancer." *International Journal of Cancer* 110(2):271–277; 2004.

"Folate and B6 from food or supplements shown to reduce heart disease risk." February 9, 2004. http://ProHealthNetwork.com.

Gallia, K., Althoff, S., and Nachatelo, M. "Blueberries fight bladder infections." *Natural Health,* April 1999, p. 24.

Grant, W. B. "The role of milk and sugar in heart disease." *American Journal of Natural Medicine* 5(9): 19–23; 1998.

Halterman, J. S., Kaczorowski, J. M., Aligne, C. A., et al. "Iron deficiency and cognitive achievement among school-aged children and adolescents in the United States. *Pediatrics* 107:1381–1386; 2001.

Handa, K., and Kreiger, N. "Diet patterns and the risk of renal cell carcinoma." *Public Health Nutrition* 5(6):757–767; 2002.

Hibbein, J. R. "Essential fatty acids predict biomarkers of aggression and depression." *PUFA Newsletter* 1(2):2.

Hornyak, M., Voderholzer, U., Hohagen, F., Berger, M., and Riemann, D. "Magnesium therapy for periodic leg movements–related insomnia and restless legs syndrome: an open pilot study." *Sleep* 21(5):501–505; 1998.

Hsieh, C. Y., Santell, R. C., Haslam, S. Z., and Helferich, W. G. "Estrogenic effects of genistein on the growth of estrogen receptor–positive human breast cancer (MCF-7) cells in vitro and in vivo." *Cancer Research,* September 1, 1998, pp. 3833–3838.

Hu, F. B., "Frequent nut consumption and risk of coronary heart disease in women." *British Medical Journal* 317:1341–1345; 1998.

Huang, C., Huang, Y., Li, J., Hu, W., Aziz, R., et al. "Inhibition of benzo(a)pyrene diol-epoxide-induced transactivation of activated protein 1 and nuclear factor kappaB by black raspberry extracts." *Cancer Research,* December 1, 2002, pp. 6857–6863.

Jenkins, D. J., Kendall, C. W., Marchie, A., Fulkner, D. A., Wong, J. M., et al. "Effects of a dietary portfolio of cholesterol-lowering foods vs. lovastatin on serum lipids and C-reactive protein." *Journal of the American Medical Association,* July 23, 2003, pp. 502–510.

Jenkins, D. J., Kendall, C. W., Marchie, A., Parker, T. L., Connelly, P. W., et al. "Dose response of almonds on coronary heart disease risk factors: blood lipids, oxidized low-density lipoproteins, lipoprotein(a), homocysteine, and pulmonary nitric oxide: a randomized, controlled, crossover trial. *Circulation,* September 10, 2002, pp. 1327–1332.

Jepson, R., Mihaljevic, L., and Craig, J. "Cranberries for preventing urinary tract infection." *Cochrane Database System Review* 2:2; 2004.

Kandiah, J. "Impact of tofu or tofu + orange juice on hematological indices of lacto-ovo vegetarian females." *Plant Foods and Human Nutrition,* Spring 2002, pp. 197–204.

Kane, E. A. "Clear up your UTI." http://Letsliveonline.com. July 2001, pp. 76–79.

Key, T. J., Allen, N. E., Spencer, E. A., and Travis, R. C. "Nutrition and breast cancer." *Breast* 12(6):412–416; 2003.

Klipstein-Grobusch, K., Grobbee, D. E., den Breeijen, J. H., Boeing, H., Hofman, A., and Witteman, J. C. "Dietary iron and risk of myocardial infarction in the Rotterdam Study. *American Journal of Epidemiology* 149(5):412–418; 1999.

Kodama, N., Komuta, K., and Nanba, H. "Can maitake MD-fraction aid cancer patients." *Alternative Medicine Review,* June 2002, pp. 236–239.

Lee, K. A., et al. "Folate, iron and restless legs syndrome." *Journal of Women's Health and Gender-Based Medicine* 10(4):335–431; 2001.

Leibel, R. L., et al., "Dieting: your metabolism fights weight loss." *New England Journal of Medicine,* March 1995, pp. 621–624.

Lian, R., Chen, M. R., and Xu, S. "Effect of dandi tablet on blood lipids and sex hormones in women of postmenopausal stage." *Zhongguo Zhong Xi Yi Jie He Za Zhi,* August 2003, pp. 593–595.

Lies, A. D., Roach, A. K., Sparks, K. C., Marquart, L., D'Agostino, R. B., Jr., and Mayer-Davis, E. J., "Whole-grain intake and insulin sensitivity: the Insulin Resistance Atherosclerosis Study." *American Journal of Clinical Nutrition.* November 2003, pp. 965–971.

Lipski, L. "Nutrition basics for women." http://www.womentowomen.com.

Lombardi-Boccia, G., Lucarini, M., Lanzi, S., Aguzzi, A., and Cappelloni, M. "Nutrients and antioxidant molecules in yellow plums (*Prunus domestica* L.). From conventional and organic productions: a comparative study." *Journal of Agricultural and Food Chemistry,* January 14, 2004, pp. 90–94.

"Long-lasting energy." http://Letsliveonline.com. February 2004, p. 36.

Malaveille, C., Hautefeuille, A., Pignatelli, B., Talaska, G., Vineis, P., and Bartsch, H. "Dietary phenolics as anti-mutagens and inhibitors of tobacco-related DNA addiction in the urothelium of smokers." *Carcinogenesis,* October 1996, pp. 2193–2200.

Mandel, S., Weinreb, O., Amit, T., and Youdim, M. B. "Cell signaling pathways in the neuroprotective actions of the green tea polyphenol (-)-epigallocatechin-3-gallate: implications for neurodegenerative diseases." *Neurochemistry,* March 2004, pp. 1555–1569.

Manz, M., and Susilo, R. "Therapy of cardiac arrhythmias. Clinical significance of potassium- and magnesium aspartate in arrhythmias." *Fortschritte der Medizin* 120(1):11–15; 2002.

Mattisson, I., Wirfalt, E., Johansson, U., Gullberg, B., Olsson, H., and Bergland, G. "Intakes of plant foods, fibre and fat and risk of breast cancer—a prospective study in the Malmo Diet and cancer cohort." *British Journal of Cancer.* January 12, 2004, pp. 122–127.

Mattisson, I., Wirfalt, E., Wallstrom, P., Gullberg, B., Olsson, H., and Berglund, G. "High fat and alcohol intakes are risk factors of postmenopausal breast cancer: a prospective study from the Malmo diet and cancer cohort." *International Journal of Cancer* 110(4): 589–597.

McLean, R.R., Jacques, D.F. Selhub, J., Tucker, K.L., Samelson, Broe, K.E., Hannan, M.T., Cupples, L.A., and Kiel, O.P. "Honocysteine as a predictive factor for hip fracture in older persons." *New England Journal of Medicine* 13(20):2042–2049; 2004.

McSorley, P.T., Young, I.S., Bell, P.M., Fee, J.P.H., and McCance, D.R. "Vitamin C improves endothelial function in healthy estrogen-deficient postmenopausal women." *Climacteric* 6(3): 238–247; 2003.

Mesina, M., and Hughes, C. "Efficacy of soyfoods and soybean isoflavone supplements for alleviating menopausal symptoms is positively related to initial hot flush frequency." *Journal of Medicinal Foods.* Spring 2003, pp. 1–11.

Muhlbauer, R.C., Lozano, A., and Reinli, A. "Onion and a mixture of vegetables, salads, and herbs affect bone resorption in the rat by a mechanism independent of their base excess." *Journal Bone and Mineral Research,* July 17, 2002, pp. 1230–1236.

Muti, P., Awad, A. B., Schunemann, H., Fink, C. S., Hovey, L., et al. "A plant food–based diet modifies the serum beta-sitosterol concentration in hyperandrogenic postmenopausal women." *Nutrition,* December 2003, pp. 4252–4255.

Nagata, C., Takatsuka, N., Kawakami, N, and Shimizu, H. "Soy product intake and hot flashes in Japanese women: results from a community-based prospective study." *American Journal of Epidemiology.* April 2001, pp. 790–793.

Nesbitt, G. H., Freeman, L. M., and Hannah, S. S. "Effect of n-3 fatty acid ratio and dose on clinical manifestations, plasma fatty acids and inflammatory mediators in dogs with pruritis." *Veterinary Dermatology.* April 2003, pp. 67–74.

Nikander, E., Metsa-Heikkila, M., Ylikorkala, O., and Tiitinen, A. "Effects of phytoestrogens on bone turnover in post-menopausal women with a history of breast cancer." *Journal of Clinical Endocrinology and Metabolism,* March 2004, pp. 1207–1212.

"Omega-3 fatty acids: Good for the heart, and (maybe) good for the brain." http://www.sciencedaily.com/releases/2004/11/041108 024221.htm accessed 11/12/04.

Opipari, A. W., Tan, L., Boitano, A. E., Sorenson, D. R., Auroa, A., and Liu, J. R. "Resveratrol-induced autophagocytosis in ovarian cancer cells." *Cancer Research,* January 15, 2004, pp. 696–703.

Osganian, S. K., Stampfer, M. J., Rimm, E., Spiegelman, D., Hu, F. B., Manson, J. E., and Willett, W. C. "Vitamin C and risk of coronary heart disease in women." *Journal of the American College of Cardiology,* July 16, 2003, pp. 246–252.

Osganian, S. K., Stampfer, M. J., Rimm, E., Spiegelman, D., Manson, J. E., and Willett, W. C. "Dietary carotenoids and risk of coronary artery disease in women." *American Journal of Clinical Nutrition.* June 2003, pp. 1390–1399.

Parcell, S. "Sulfur in human nutrition and applications in medicine." *Alternative Medical Review,* February 2002, pp. 22–44.

Peatfield, R. C. "Relationships between food, wine, and beer-precipitated migrainous headaches." *Headache,* June 1995, pp. 355–357.

Peck, L. W., Monsen, E. R., and Ahmad, S. "Effect of three sources of long-chain fatty acids on the plasma fatty acid profile, plasma prostaglandin E2 concentrations, and pruritus symptoms in hemodialysis patients." *American Journal of Clinical Nutrition.* August 1996, pp. 210–214.

Perrig, W. J., Perrig, P., and Stahelin, H. B. "The relation between antioxidants and memory performance in the old and very old." *Journal of American Geriatric Society* 45:718–747; 1997.

Peters, S. "Menopause: a new era, new strategies offer more choices to women." *Advance for Nurse Practitioners.* July 1998, pp. 61–64.

Pettit, J. L., "Alternative medicine—soy." *Clinician Reviews,* June 2001, pp. 119–120.

Pierre, F., Tache, S., Petit, C. R., Van der Meer, R., and Corepet, D. E. "Meat and cancer: haemoglobin and haemin in low-calcium diet promote colorectal carcinogenesis at the aberrant crypt stage in rats." *Carcinogenesis* 24(10):1683–1690; 2003.

Plotnick, G. D., Corretti, M. C., Vogel, R. A., Hesslink, R., Jr., and Wise, J. A. "Effect of supplemental phytonutrients on impairment of the flow-mediated brachial artery vasoactivity after a single high-fat meal." *Journal of the American College of Cardiology,* May 21, 2003, pp. 1744–1749.

Pool-Zobol, B. L., et al. "Consumption of vegetables reduces genetic damage in humans: first results of a human intervention trial with carotenoid-rich foods." *Carcinogenesis* 18:1847–1850; 1997.

Potischman, N., Coates, R. J., Swanson, C. A., Carroll, R. J., et al. "Increased risk of early-stage breast cancer related to consumption of sweet foods among women less than age 48 in the United States." *Cancer Causes and Control* 13(10):937–946.

Potter, S. M., "Soy protein and cardiovascular disease." *Nutrition Reviews* 56(8): 231–35; 1998.

Radzikowski, C., Wietrzyk, J., Grynkiewicz, G., and Opolski, A. "Genistein: a soy isoflavone revealing a pleiotropic mechanism of action—clinical implications in the treatment and prevention of cancer." *Postepyhigieny I Medvjcyrry Doswiadczalnei,* February 27, 2004, pp. 128–139.

Rees, C. A., Bauer, J. E., Burkholder, W. J., Kennis, R. A., Dunbar, B. L., and Bigley, K. E. "Effects of dietary flax seed and sunflower seed supplementation on normal canine serum. Polyunsaturated fatty acids and skin and hair coat condition scores." *Veterinary Dermatology* April 2001, pp. 111–117.

Rosch, P., and Clark, C. C. *De-Stress, Weigh Less: A Six-Step, No-Diet Plan for Relaxing Your Way to Permanent Weight Loss.* New York: St. Martins Press, 2001.

Rose, D. P., Boyar, A. P., Cohen, C., and Strong, L. E. "Effect of low-fat diet on hormone levels in women with cystic breast disease." *Journal of the National Cancer Institute* 78(4): 623–626; 1987.

Samman, S., Sivarajah, G., Man, J. C., Ahmad, Z. I., Petocz, P., and Caterson, I. D., "A mixed fruit and vegetable concentrate increases plasma antioxidant vitamins and folate and lowers plasma homocysteine in men." *Journal of Nutrition,* July 2003, pp. 2188–2193.

Savi, L., Rainero, I., Valfre, W., Gentile, S., Lo, G. R., and Pinessi, L. "Food and headache attacks. A comparison of patients with migraine and tension-type headache." *Panminerva Medicine,* March 2002, pp. 27–31.

Simopoulos, A. P. "The traditional diet of Greece and cancer." *European Journal of Cancer Prevention* 13(3):219–230; 2004.

Slattery, M. L., Levin, T. R., Ma. K., Goldgar, D., Holubkov, R., et al. "Family history and colorectal cancer: predictors of risk." *Cancer Causes and Control* 13(9):879–887; 2003.

Solfrizzi, V., Panza, F., Tones, F., Mastroianna, F., Del Parigi, A., Venezia, A., and Capurso, A. "A High monounsaturated fatty acids intake protects against age-related cognitive decline." *Neurology* 52(8):1563–1569; 1999.

Stone, F. "Iron helps build bones." http://www.medicinenet.com /script/main/art.asp?articlekey=26743.

Stoner, G. D., Kresty, L. A., Carlton, P. S., Siglin, J. C., and Morse, M. A. "Isothiocyanates and freeze-dried strawberries as inhibitors of esophageal cancer." *Toxicology and Science,* December 1999, pp. 85–100.

Su, K. P., Huang, S. Y., Chiu, C. C., and Shen, W. W. "Omega-3 fatty acids in major depressive disorder. *European Neuropharmacology* 13(4): 261–271; 2003.

Sun, J. "Morning/evening menopausal formula relieves menopausal symptoms: a pilot study." *Journal of Alternative and Complementary Medicine*, June 2003, pp. 403–409.

Sun, J., Chu, Y. F., Wu, X., and Liu, R. H. "Antioxidant and antiproliferative activities of common fruits." *Agricultural and Food Chemistry,* December 4, 2002, pp. 7449–7454.

Tian, Q., Miller, E. G., Ahmad, H., Tang, L., and Patil, B. S. "Differential inhibition of human cancer cell proliferation by citrus limonoids." *Nutrition and Cancer* 40(2): 180–184; 2001.

Tuomainen, T. P., Punnonen, K., Nyyssonene, K. I., and Salonen, J. T. "Association between body iron stores and the risk of acute myocardial infarction in men." *Circulation* 97(15): 1461–1466; 1998.

Tweed, V. "The latest on cancer prevention." http://Letsliveonline. com, February 2004, p. 34.

Wallace, K. "Research sheds new light on causes, potential treatment for interstitial cystitis." *News from the National Kidney Foundation of Florida,* March 1, 1995.

Whiting, S., Wood, R., and Kim, K. "Pharmacology Update: Calcium Supplementation," *Journal of American Academy of Nurse Practitioners* 9(4):187–192; 1997.

Wiklund, I. K., Mattsson, L. A., Lindgren, R., and Limoni, C. "Effects of a standardized ginseng extract on quality of life and physiological parameters in symptomatic postmenopausal women: a double-blind, placebo-controlled trial." *International Journal of Clinical and Pharmacological Research* 19(3):89–99; 1999.

Williams, D. "Sure cure for bladder and kidney infections?" *Alternatives* 1(20): 3; 1995.

Zheng, W., Dai, Q., Custer, I. J., et al. "Urinary excretion of isoflavonoids and the risk of breast cancer." *Cancer Epidemiology and Biomarkers in Prevention* 8: 35–40; 1999.

Zhou, J. R., Yu, L., Mai, Z., and Blackburn, G. L. "Combined inhibition of estrogen-dependent human breast carcinoma by soy and tea bioactive components in mice." *International Journal of Cancer,* January 1, 2004, pp. 8–14.

Chapter 5: Herbs

Aesoph, L. M. "Five remedies for restful sleep." http://Letsliveonline.com. December 2000, pp. 64–67.

Amato, P., Christophe, S., and Mellon, P. L. "Estrogenic activity of herbs commonly used as remedies for menopausal symptoms." *Menopause,* March–April 2002, pp. 145–150.

American College of Obstetricians and Gynecologists (ACOG). "Guidelines on the most popular herbal products for menopause." http://www.4woman.gov/faq/menopaus.htm.

Armanini, D., De Palo, C. B., Mattarello, M. J., Spinella, P., Zaccaria, M., et al. "Effect of licorice on the reduction of body fat mass in healthy subjects." *Journal of Endocrinological Investigation,* July 2003, pp. 646–650.

Atkinson, C., Warren, R. M., Sala, E., Dowsett, M., Dunning, A. M., et al. "Red clover–derived isoflavones and mammographic breast density: a double-blind, randomized, placebo-controlled trial." *Breast Cancer Research* 6(3):R170–179; 2004.

Baber, R. J., Templeman, C., Morton, T., Kelly, G. E., and West, L. "Randomized placebo-controlled trial of an isoflavone supplement and menopausal symptoms in women." *Climacteric* 2(2):85–92; 1999.

Bhattacharya, S. K., Bhattacharya, A., Sairam, K., and Ghosal, S. "Anxiolytic-antidepressant activity of *Withania somnifera* glycowithanolides: an experimental study." *Phytomedicine,* December 2000, pp. 464–469.

Blumenthal, M., Busse, W. R., Goldberg, A., et al. *The Complete German Commission E Monographs: Therapeutic Guide to Herbal Medicine,* 1st edition. Austin, TX: American Botanical Council, 1998.

Brewer, S. "Sex treatment." *Greatlife,* April 1998, pp. 32–35.

Burdette, J. E., Liu, J., Chen, S. N., Fabricant, D. S., Piersen, C. E., et al. "Black cohosh acts as a mixed competitive ligand and partial agonist of the serotonin receptor." *Journal of Agricultural and Food Chemistry,* September 10, 2003, pp. 5661–5670.

Cass, H. "Kava: Is it safe?" http://www.cassmd.com/library/Kava. warnings.html.

Charmasiri, M. G., Jayakody, J. R., Galhena, G., Liyanage, S. S., and Ratnasooriya, W. D. "Anti-inflammatory and analgesic activities of mature fresh leaves of *Vitex negundo*." *Journal of Ethnopharmacology,* August 2003, pp. 199–206.

Clootre, D. I., "Kava Kava: examining new reports of toxicity." *Toxicology Letter,* 150(1):85–96, 2004.

Cuccinelli, J. H. "Ginkgo biloba." *Clinician Reviews* 9(8):93–95, 1999.

Dailey, R. K., Neale, A. V., Northrup, J., West, P., and Schwartz, K. L. "Herbal product use and menopause symptom relief in primary care patients: a MetroNet study." *Journal of Women's Health,* September 2003, pp. 633–641.

de Sousa, A. C., Alviano, D. S., Blank, A. F., Alves, P. B., Alviano, C. S., et al. "*Melissa officinalis* L. Essential oil: antitumoral and antioxidant activities." *Journal of Pharmaceutical Pharmacology*, May 2004, pp. 677–681.

Dhingra, D., Parle, M., and Kulkarni, S. K. "Memory enhancing activity of *Glycyrrhiza glabra* in mice." *Journal of Ethnopharmacology*, April 2004, pp. 361–364.

Diener, H. C., Rahifs, V. W., and Danesch, U. "The first placebo-controlled trial of a special butterbur root extract for the prevention of migraine: reanalysis of efficacy criteria." *European Neurology*, January 28, 2004, pp. 89–97.

Dog, T. L., Powell, K. L., and Weisman, S. M. "Critical evaluation of the safety of Cimicifuga racemosa in menopause symptom relief." *Menopause* 10(4):299–313; 2003.

Elkins, M. H. "The lady in red (clover that is)." http://Letslive online.com. August 2001, pp. 79–81.

Gertz, H. J., and Kiefer, M. "Review about ginkgo biloba special extract Egb 761 (ginkgo)." *Current Pharmaceutical Design* 10(3):261–264; 2004.

Gulcin, I., Kufrevioglu, O. I., Oktay, M., and Buyukokuroglu, M. E. "Antioxidant, antimicrobial, antiulcer, and analgesic activities of nettle (*Urtica dioica* L.)." *Journal of Ethnopharmacology* 90(2–3):205–215; 2004.

Hadley, S., and Petry, J. J. "Valerian." *American Family Physician*, April 2003, pp. 1755–1758.

Hallam, K. T., Olver, J. S., McGrath, C., and Norman, T. R. "Comparative cognitive and psychomotor effects of single doses of *Valeriana officianalis* and triazolam in healthy volunteers." *Human Psychopharmacology*, December 2003, pp. 619–625.

Jeri, A. R. "The effect of isoflavones phytoestrogens in relieving hot flushes in Peruvian postmenopausal women." Paper presented at the 9th International Menopause Society World Congress, October 19, 1999, Yokahama, Japan.

Jo, E. H., Hong, H. D., Ahn, N. C., Jung, J. W., Yang, S. R., et al. "Modulations of the Bcl-2/Bax family were involved in the chemopreventive effects of licorice root (*Glycyrrhiza uralensis* Fisch) in MCF-7 human breast cancer cell." *Journal of Agricultural and Food Chemistry* 52(6):1715–1719; 2004.

Kennedy, D. O., Wake, G., Saveley, S., Tildesley, N. T., Perry, E. K., et al. "Modulation of mood and cognitive performance following acute administration of single doses of *Melissa officinalis* (lemon balm) with human CNS nicotinic and muscarinic receptor-binding properties." *Neuropsychopharmacology* 28 (10):1871–1881; 2003.

Kliger, B. "Black cohosh." *American Family Physician,* July 1, 2003, pp. 114–116.

Kobayashi, Y., Nakano, Y., Inayama, K., Sakai, A., and Kamiya, T. "Dietary intake of the flower extracts of German chamomile (*Matricaria recutita* L.) inhibited compound 48/80-induced itch-scratch responses in mice." *Phytomedicine,* November 2003, pp. 657–664.

Lehrl, S. "Clinical efficacy of kava extract WS 1490 in sleep disturbances associated with anxiety disorders. Results of a multicenter, randomized, placebo-controlled, double-blind clinical trial." *Journal of Affective Disorders* 78(2):101–110; 2004.

Lieberman, S. "A review of the effectiveness of black cohosh for the symptoms of menopause." *Journal of Women's Health* 7:525–529; 2001.

Liske, E. "Therapeutic efficacy and safety of *Cimicifuga racemos* (black cohosh) for gynecologic disorders." *Advanced Therapeutics* 15:45–53; 1998.

Liske, E. "Therapy of climacteric complaints with *Cimicifuga racemosa* (black coshosh): herbal medicine with clinically proven evidence." *Menopause* 5:250; 1998.

Liu, J., Burdette, J. E., Xu, H., Gu, C., van Breemen, R. B., et al. "Evaluation of estrogenic activity of plant extracts for the potential treatment of menopausal symptoms." *Journal of Agricultural and Food Chemistry,* May 2001, pp. 2472–2479.

Lupu, R., Mehmi, I., Atlas, E., Tsai, M. S. Pisha, E., et al. "Black cohosh, a menopausal remedy, does not have estrogenic activity and does not promote breast cancer cell growth." *International Journal of Oncology,* November 2003, pp. 1407–1412.

Mackey, B. T. "Herbal therapies." In C. C. Clark, editor-in-chief, *Encyclopedia of Complementary Health Practice.* New York: Springer, pp. 382–385.

Mauskop, A., Grossman, W., Schmmidramst, et al. "*Petasites hydratus* (butterbur root) extract is effective in the prophylaxis of migraines: results of a randomized, double-blind trial." *Headache* 40:420; 2000.

Mishra, L. C., Singh, B. B., and Dagenais, S. "Scientific basis for the therapeutic use of *Withania somnifera* (ashwagandha): a review." *Alternative Medicine Review* 5(4):334–346; 2000.

North American Menopause Society. "Treatment of menopause-associated vasomotor symptoms: position statement of the North American Menopause Society." *Menopause,* 11(1): 11–33; 2004.

Northrup, C. "Menopause." *Complementary and Alternative Therapies in Primary Care,* December 1997, pp. 921–948.

Petit, J. L. "Black cohosh." *Clinican Reviews* 10(4):117–119; 2000.

Powles, T. "Isoflavones and women's health." *Breast Cancer Research* 6(3):140–142; 2004.

Ramsey, L. A., Ross, B. S., and Fischer, R. G. "Management of menopause." *Advance for Nurse Practitioners,* May 1999, pp. 27–30.

Thomsen, M., and Schmidt, M. "Hepatotoxicity from *Cimicifuga racemosa*? Recent Australian case report not sufficiently substantiated." *Journal of Alternative and Complementary Medicine* 9(3):337–340; 2003.

Tzingounis, M. A. "Estriol in the management of the menopause." *Journal of the American Medical Association* 239:1638–1644; 1978.

Van deWeijer, P. H., and Barentsen, R. "Isoflavones from red clover (Promensil) significantly reduce menopausal hot flush symptoms compared with placebo. *Naturttis* 42(3):187–193; 2002.

Wang, X., Wu, J., Chiba, H., Umegaki, K., Yamada, K., and Ishimi, Y. "*Puerariae radix* prevents bone loss in ovariectomized mice." *Bone Mineral Metabolism* 21(5):269–275; 2003.

Weil, A. "Dong quai: The female ginseng." *Self-Healing,* February 1998, p. 2.

Weil, A. "Coping with hot flashes and insomnia." *Self-Healing,* July 1998, p. 3.

Yuan, C. S., Mehendale, S., Xiao, Y., Aung, H. H., Xie, J. T., et al. "The gamma-aminobutyric acidergic effects of valerian and valerenic acid on rat brainstem neuronal activity." *Anesthesia and Analgesia*, February 2004, pp. 353–358.

Ziegler, G., Ploch, M., Miettinen-Baumann, A., and Collet, W. "Efficacy and tolerability of valerian extract LI 156 compared with oxazepam in the treatment of non-organic insomnia—a randomized, double-blind, comparative clinical study." *European Journal of Medical Research*, November 2002, pp. 480–486.

Chapter 6: Environmental Actions

Aesoph, L. M. "Five remedies for restful sleep." http://Letsliveonline. com. December 2000, pp. 64–67.

Boisnic, S., Branchet-Gumila, M. C., and Coutanceau, C. "Inhibitory effect of oatmeal extract oligomer on vasoactive intestinal peptide-induced inflammation in surviving human skin." *International Journal of Tissue Reactions* 25(2):41–46; 2003.

Brewer, S. "Sex treatment." *GreatLife,* April 1998, pp. 32–35.

Chakalis, E., and Lowe, G. "Positive effects of subliminal stimulation on memory." *Perceptual Motor Skills* 74(3, Pt. 1): 956–958; 1992.

Dolby, V. "Nature's aphrodisiacs." *Let's Live,* February 1998, pp. 67–71.

Dolby, V. "Maximize your memory: top 10 ways to build a better brain." *Let's Live,* June 1998, pp. 35–39.

Franklin, B. "Is any estrogen too much?" *Let's Live,* March 1996, pp. 16–18.

Goldstein, L. "Using baking soda to relieve a painful problem." *The Herald-Sun,* July 29, 2001, p. 16.

Graedon, J., and Graedon, T. "A new use for ginkgo biloba?" *St. Petersburg Times,* November 3, 1998, p. 3D.

Higg, D. "Aromatherapy for lovers: sexy scents." *Let's Live,* April 1998, pp. 58–64.

Landis, B. "Fighting vaginal dryness without estrogen." *The Clinical Advisor,* May 2004, p. 59.

Love, S. "What can I do for vaginal dryness?" http://www.SusanLoveMD.org.

Martin, N. "Multitasking makes you sick." *Organic Style,* November/December 2003, pp. 55–61.

Moneysmith, M. "Revitalize romance." *GreatLife,* February 2002, pp. 34–36.

National Kidney Foundation of Florida. "Studies reveal new hope for women who suffer from chronic UTIs." (407) 894-7325.

Noonan, P. J. "Skin: makeup makes women face more itches." *USA Weekend,* May 14–16, 2004, p. 13.

Redeker, N. S., and Nadolski, N. "Treating insomnia in primary care." *American Journal for Nurse Practitioners* 8(3):61–66; 2004.

Rodale Press. "Great gifts can be found at the health food store." *The Herald-Sun,* December 15, 2002, p. 12.

Rogers, S. A. "Is your office toxic?" http://letsliveonline.com, pp. 74–75.

Schmidt, L. A., Fox, N. A., Goldberg, M. C., Smith, C. C., and Schulkin, J. "Effects of acute prednisone administration on memory, attention, and emotion in healthy human adults." *Psychoneuroendocrinology* 24(4):461–483; 1999.

Staab, A. M. "Breaking an unhealthy habit." *Clinician Reviews* 13(7):24; 2003.

U.S. Department of Health and Human Services. "You can quit smoking." ISSN 1530-6402, U.S. Government Printing Office, 2000.

Vanderwater-Piercy, K. "Freedom from smoking: succeeding where others fail." *Advance for Nurse Practitioners,* October 1995, pp. 41–52.

Weiner, E. "Better memory." *Bottom Line Personal,* March 1, 1994, p. 5.

Williams, D. "Fluoridated water makes matters worse." *Alternatives,* February 1999, p. 160.

Woodward, S. "Insomnia: better than drugs." *Women's Health Advocate,* November 1998, p. 3.

Chapter 7: Exercise

Bailey, D. M., Young, I. S., McEneny, J., Lawrenson, L., Kim, J., et al. "Regulation of free radical outflow from an isolated muscle bed in exercising humans." *American Journal of Physiology and Heart Circulation Physiology* 287(4):H1689–1699; 2004.

Chan, K., Qin, L., Lau, M., Woo, J., Au, S., et al. "A randomized prospective study of the effects of tai chi chun exercise on bone mineral density in postmenopausal women." *Archives of Physical Medicine and Rehabilitation* 85(5):717–722; 2004.

Chang, S. T. *The Complete System of Self-Healing: Internal Exercises.* San Francisco: Tao Publishing, 1991.

Cleary, M. A., Kimura, I. F., Sitler, M. R., and Kendrick, Z. V. "Temporal pattern of the repeated bout effect of eccentric exercise on delayed-onset muscle soreness." *Journal of Athletic Training* 37(1):32–36; 2002.

Corna, S., Nardone, A., Prestinari, A., Galante, M., Grasso, M., et al. "Comparison of Cawthorne-Cooksey exercises and sinusoidal support surface translations to improve balance in patients with unilateral vestibular deficit." *Archives of Physical Medicine and Rehabilitation* 84(8):1173–1184; 2003.

Gemben, D. A., Fetters, N. L., Bemben, M. G., Nabavi, N., and Koh, E. T. "Musculoskeletal responses to high- and low-intensity resistance training in early postmenopausal women." *Medical Science and Sport Exercise* 32(11):1949–1957; 2000.

Guthrie, J. R., Taffee, J. R., Lehert, P., Burger, H. G., and Dennerstine, L. "Association between hormonal changes at menopause and the risk of a coronary event: a longitudinal study." *Menopause* 11(3):315–322; 2004.

Holmes, M. "Exercise improves chances of survival." Presented at the American Association for Cancer Research, Orlando, March 29, 2004.

Hull, A. R. "Urinary incontinence increasing among postmenopausal women: nonsurgical treatments often helpful." News Release, National Kidney Foundation, New York; (800) 622-9010.

Jenkins, D. J., Kendall, C. W., Marchie, A., Parker, J. L., Connelly, P. W., et al. "Dose response of almonds on coronary heart disease risk factors." *Circulation* 66(11):1314–1332; 2002.

Johnson, K. "Exercise improves libido in menopausal women." *Clinical Psychiatry News,* December 2003, p. 50.

Kaminsky, L. "Walk to keep the holiday pounds off." Ball State University News Release, December 9, 2003. http://www.beu.edu/news.

Kando, J. *The Natural Face Book.* Hammersmith, London: Thorsons, 1991.

Kemmler, W., Lauber, D., Weineck, J., Hensen, J., Kalender, W., et al. "Benefits of 2 years of intense exercise on bone density, physical fitness, and blood lipids in early postmenopausal osteopenic women: results of the Erlangen Fitness Osteoporosis Prevention Study (EFOPS)." *Archives of Internal Medicine* 164(10):1084–1091; 2004.

Kerr, D., Ackland, T., Maslen, B., Morton, A., and Prince, R. "Resistance training over 2 years increases bone mass in calcium-replete postmenopausal women." *Journal of Bone and Mineral Research* 16(1):175–181; 2001.

Kessel, B. "Hip fracture prevention in postmenopausal women." *Obstetrics and Gynecology Survey* 59(6):446–455; 2004.

Knaster, M. *Discovering the Body's Wisdom.* New York: Bantam Books, 1996.

Koseoglu, E., Akboyraz, A., Soyuer, A., and Ersoy, A. O. "Aerobic exercise and plasma beta endorphin levels in patients with migrainous headache without aura." *Cephalgia* 23(10):962–966; 2003.

Kozora, E., Tran, Z. V., and Make, B. "Neurobehavioral improvement after brief rehabilitation in patients with chronic obstructive pulmonary disease." *Journal of Cardiopulmonary Rehabilitation* 22(6):416–430; 2002.

Lavie, C. V., and Milani, R. V. "Impact of aging on hostility in coronary patients and effects of cardiac rehabilitation and exercise training in elderly persons." *American Journal of Geriatric Cardiology* 13(3):125–130; 2004.

Marshall, L. *Keep Up with Yoga.* New York: Sterling Publishing Company, 1989.

Mastrangelo, R., and Gerchufsky, M. "Headache." *Advance for Nurse Practitioners*, December 1994, pp. 9–11.

Mauskop, A. "Alternative therapies in headache. Is there a role?" *Medical Clinics of North America* 85(4):1077–1084; 2001.

McTiernan, A., Kooperberg, C., White, E., Wilcox, S., Coates, R., et al. "Recreational physical activity and the risk of breast cancer in postmenopausal women: the Women's Health Initiative Cohort Study." *Journal of the American Medical Association* 290(10): 1331–1336; 1989.

"Menopause: sweat out your symptoms." http://www.bssjconnec tions.com/women/article.asp?L=1833&A-1455.

Messier, S. P., Loeser, R. F., Miller, G. D., Morgan, T. M., Rejeski, W. J., et al. "Exercise and dietary weight loss in overweight and obese older adults with knee osteoarthritis: the Arthritis, Diet, and Activity Promotion Trial." *Arthritis and Rheumatology* 50(5): 1501–1510; 2004.

Meston, C. M., and Gorzalka, B. B. "Differential effects of sympathetic activation on sexual arousal in sexually dysfunctional and functional women." *Journal of Abnormal Psychology* 105(4):583–591; 1996.

Nieman, L. K. "Management of surgically hypogonadal patients unable to take sex hormone replacement therapy." *Endocrinology and Metabolic Clinics of North America* 32(2): 325–336; 2003.

North American Menopause Society. "Consider other treatments for mild menopause symptoms." *Menopause* 11:11–31; 2004.

Oldervoll, L. M., Kaasa, S., Knobel, H., and Loge, J. H. "Exercise reduces fatigue in chronic fatigued Hodgkin's disease survivors—results from a pilot study." *European Journal of Cancer* 39(1):57–63; 2003.

Patel, A. V., Press, M. F., Meeske, K., Calie, E. E., and Bernstein, L. "Lifetime recreational exercise and risk of breast carcinoma in situ." http://www.weightlossresource.com/library/print.cfm?ID=1641.

Pearson, D. "Weight training helps the body look younger." University Communications, Muncie, IN. June 2004. http://www.bsu.edu/newsucomm@bsu.edu.

Perry, R. *Reverse the Aging Process of Your Face*. Garden City Park, NY: Avery Publishing Group, 1995.

Richardson, M. R. "Current perspectives in polycystic ovary syndrome." *American Family Physician* 68(4):697–704; 2003.

Satoh, T., Sakurai, I., Miyagi, K., and Hohshaku, Y. "Walking exercise and improved neuropsychological functioning in elderly patients with cardiac disease." *Journal of Internal Medicine* 238(5):423–428; 1995.

Schlosberg, S. "Pain busters." http://www.aarpmagazine.com. January–February 2004.

Schutte, S., and Doghramji, K. "Eyes wide open: update on sleep disorders." *The Clinical Advisor*, February 2003, pp. 17–27.

Serizawa, K. *Massage: The Oriental Method.* San Francisco: Japan Publications, 1972.

Stean, J. *Yoga, Youth & Reincarnation.* Virginia Beach: A.R.E. Press, 1997.

Teoman, N., Ozcan, A., and Acar, B. "The effect of exercise on physical fitness and quality of life in postmenopausal women." *Maturitas* 47(1):71–77; 2004.

Tworoger, S. S., Yasui, Y., Vitiello, M. V., Schwartz, R. S., Ulrich, C. M., et al. "Effects of a yearlong moderate-intensity exercise and a stretching intervention on sleep quality in post-menopausal women." *Sleep* 26(7):830–836; 2003.

Ueda, M., and Tokunaga, M. "Effects of exercise experienced in the life stages on climacteric symptoms for females." *Journal of Physiological Anthropology and Applied Human Science* (19(4):181–189; 2000.

Wegge, J. K., Roberts, C. K., Ngo, T. H., and Barnard, R. J. "Effect of diet and exercise intervention on inflammatory and adhesion molecules in postmenopausal women on hormone replacement therapy and at risk for coronary artery disease." *Metabolism* 53(3): 377–381; 2004.

Yamamoto, S., and McCarty, P. *The Shiatsu Handbook: A Guide to the Traditional Art of Shiatsu Acupressure.* Garden City Park, NY: Avery Publishing Group, 1996.

Zelinski, M. R., Muenchow, M., Wallig, M. A., Horn, P. L., and Woods, J. A. "Exercise delays allogeneic tumor growth and reduces intratumoral inflammation and vascularization." *Journal of Applied Physiology* 96(6):2249–2256. Epub March 12, 2004.

Chapter 8: Other Stress Reduction and Healing Measures

Bakke, A.C., Purtzer, M.Z., and Newton, P. "The effect of hypnotic-guided imagery on psychological well-being and immune function in patients with prior breast cancer." *Journal of Psychosomatic Research,* December 2002, pp. 1131–1137.

Burns, D.D. *The Feeling Good Handbook.* New York: Penguin Group, 1990.

China Sports Magazine. *The Wonders of Qigong.* Wayfarer Publications, 1985.

Enqvist, B., von Konow, L., and Bystedt, H. "Pre- and perioperative suggestion in maxillofacial surgery: effects on blood loss and recovery." *International Journal of Clinical Experimental Hypnosis* 43(3):284–295; 1995.

Floyd, M., Scogin, F., McKendree-Smith, N.L., Floyd, D.L., and Rokke, P.D. "Cognitive therapy for depression: a comparison of individual psychotherapy and bibliotherapy for depressed older adults." *Behavior Modification* 28(2):197–318; 2004.

Fuchs, K. "Therapy of vaginismus by hypnotic desensitization." *American Journal of Obstetrics and Gynecology* 137(1):1–7; 1980.

Ganz, P.A., Greendale, G.A., Peterson, L., Bibecchi, L., Kahn, B., and Belin, T.R. "Managing menopausal symptoms in breast cancer survivors." *Journal of the National Cancer Institute* 92(13): 1001–1064; 2000.

Ginandes, C.S., and Rosenthal, D.J. "Using hypnosis to accelerate the healing of bone fractures: a randomized controlled pilot study." *Alternative Therapies* 5(2):67–75; 1999.

Glavind, K., Mouritsen, A.L., and Lose, G. *Ugeskrift for laeger* 160(2):157–162; 1998.

Gruzelier, J.H. "A review of the impact of hypnosis, relaxation, guided imagery and individual differences on aspects of immunity and health." *Stress* 5(2):147–63; 2002.

Hammond, D. C. "Treatment of chronic fatigue with neurofeedback and self-hypnosis." *NeuroRehabilitation* 16(4): 295–300; 2001.

Kelly, A. E., Sullivan, P., Fawcett, J., and Samarel, N. "Therapeutic touch, quiet time and dialogue: perceptions of women with breast cancer." *Oncology Nursing Forum*, May 2004, pp. 625–631.

King, L. "Gain without pain? Expressive writing and self-regulation." In S. J. Lepore and J. M. Smyth (Eds.), *The Writing Cure: How Expressive Writing Promotes Health and Emotional Well-Being.* American Psychological Association, pp. 119–134; 2002.

King, L. "The health benefits of writing about life goals." *Personality and Social Psychology Bulletin* 27: 198–207; 2001.

Kistler, A., Mariauzouls, C., Wyler, F., Bircher, A. J., and Wyler-Harper, J. "Autonomic responses to suggestions for cold and warmth in hypnosis." *Research in Complementary and Classical Natural Medicine* 6(2): 10–14; 1999.

LaBaw, W. "The use of hypnosis with hemophilia." *Psychiatric Medicine* 10(4): 89–98; 1992.

Lee, M. S., Kim, H. J., and Moon, S. R. "Qigong reduced blood pressure and catecholamine levels of patients with essential hypertension." *International Journal of Neuroscience* 113(12): 1691–1701; 2003.

Lucero, M. A., and McCloskey, W. W. "Alternatives to estrogen for the treatment of hot flashes." *Annals of Pharmacotherapy* July–August 1997, pp. 915–917.

Rucklidge, J. J., and Saunders, D. "Hypnosis in a case of long-standing idiopathic itch." *Psychosomatic Medicine* 61(3): 355–358; 1999.

Seskevich, J. E., Crater, S. W., Lane, J. D., and Krucof, M. W. "Beneficial effects of noetic therapies on mood before percutaneous intervention for unstable coronary syndromes." *Nursing Research,* March–April 2004, pp. 116–121.

Shenefelt, P. D. "Biofeedback, cognitive-behavioral in methods, and hypnosis in dermatology: is it all in your mind?" *Dermatological Therapy* 16(2):114–122; 2003.

Smith, M. T., and Neubauer, D. N. "Cognitive behavior therapy for chronic insomnia." *Clinical Cornerstone* 5(3):28–40; 2003.

Stiefel, F., and Stagno, D. "Management of insomnia in patients with chronic pain conditions." *Central Nervous System Drugs* 18(5):285–96; 2004.

Stradling, J., Roberts, D., Wilson, A., and Lovelock, F. "Controlled trial of hypnotherapy for weight loss in patients with obstructive sleep apnea." *International Journal of Obesity and Related Metabolic Disorders* 22(3):278–281; 1998.

Wijma, K., Melin, A., Nedstrand, E., and Hammar, M. "Treatment of menopausal symptoms with applied relaxation: a pilot study." *Journal of Behavioral Therapy and Experimental Psychiatry* 28(4):251–261; 1997.

Williams, D. "Are you switched?" *Alternatives* 2(6):2–3; 1987.

Winocur, E., Gavish, A., Emodi-Perlman, A., Halachmi, M., and Eli, L. "Hypnorelaxation as treatment for myofascial pain disorder: a comparative study." *Oral Surgery, Oral Medicine, Oral Pathology, Oral Radiology and Endodentistry* 93(4): 429–434; 2002.

Wolsko, P. M., Eisenberg, D. M., Davis, R. B., and Phillips, R. S. "Use of mind-body medical therapies." *Journal of General and Internal Medicine*, January 2004, pp. 43–50.

Younus, J., Simpson, I., Collins, A., and Wang, X. "Mind control of menopause." *Women's Health Issues* 13(2):74–78; 2003.

Chapter 9: Relationships

Avis, N. E., Crawford, S., and Manuel, J. "Psychosocial problems among younger women with breast cancer." *Psychooncology*, May 2004, pp. 295–308.

Clark, C. C. "Positive relationship building." *Wellness Practitioner.* New York: Springer, 1996.

Danaci, A. E., Oruc, S., Adiguzel, H., Yildirim., Y., and Aydemir, O. "Relationship of sexuality with psychological and hormonal features in the menopausal period." *West Indian Medical Journal,* March 2003, pp. 27–30.

Dennerstein, L., Dudley, E., Guthrie, J., and Barrett-Connor, E. "Life satisfaction, symptoms, and the menopausal transition." *Medscape Women's Health,* July–August 2000, p. E4.

Gallo, L. C., Truxel, W. M., Matthews, K. A., and Kuller, L. H. "Marital status and quality in middle-aged women: associations with levels and trajectories of cardiovascular risk factors." *Health Psychology,* September 2003, pp. 453–463.

Chapter 10: Changes, Demands, and Supports

Clark, C. C. (Ed.). *The Encyclopedia of Complementary Health Practice.* New York: Springer, 1999.

Chapter 11: Finding and Working with the Right Practitioner

Bertakis, K. D., Franks, P., and Azari, R. "Effects of physician gender on patient satisfaction." *Journal of the American Medical Women's Association,* Spring 2003, pp. 69–75.

Boon, H., Stewart, M., Kennard, M. A., and Guimond, J. "Visiting family physicians and naturopathic practitioners. Comparing patient–practitioner interactions." *Canadian Family Physician* 49:1481–1487; 2003.

Clark, C. C. (Ed.). *The Encyclopedia of Complementary Health Practice.* New York: Springer, 1999.

Cooper, L. A., Roter, E. L., Johnson, R. L., Ford, D. E., Steinwachs, D. M., and Power, N. R. "Patient-centered communication, ratings, of care, and concordance of patient and physician race." *Annals of Internal Medicine* 139(11):907–915; 2003.

Flocke, S. A., Miller, W. L., and Crabtree, B. F. "Relationships between physician practice style, patient satisfaction, and attributes of primary care." *Journal of Family Practice* 51 (10):835–840; 2002.

Kinchen, K. S., Cooper, L. A., Levine, D., Wang, N. Y., and Powe, N. R. "Referral of patients to specialists: factors affecting choice of specialist by primary care physicians." *American Family Medicine* 2(3):245–252; 2004.

Pinkerton, J. A., and Bush, H. A. "Nurse practitioners and physicians: patients' perceived health and satisfaction with care." *Journal of the American Academy of Nurse Practitioners* 12(6):211–217; 2000.

Rainer, S., Daughtridge, R., and Sloane, P. D. "Physician–patient communication in the primary care office: a systematic review." *Journal of the American Board of Family Practice* 15(1):25–38; 2002.

Roter, D. L., and Hall, J. A. Physician gender and patient-centered communication: a critical review of empirical research." *Annual Review of Public Health* 25:497–519; 2004.

Roter, D. L., Stewart, M., Putnam, S. M., Lipkin, M., Jr., Stiles, W., and Inui, T. S. "Communication patterns of primary care physicians." *Journal of the American Medical Association* 277(4):350–356; 1997.

Street, R. L., Jr., Krupat, E., Bella, R. A., Kravitz, R. L., and Haidet, P. "Beliefs about control in the physician–patient relationship: effect on communication in medical encounters." *Journal of General Internal Medicine* 18(8):609–616; 2003.

Chapter 12: Putting It All Together: Your Menopause Success Plan

Menopause at Bellaonline.com Web site. http://Menopause. bellaonline.com.

INDEX

saliva test, 60
surgical preparation, 65
yam creams, 55
Nurse's Study and heart disease, 97

oatmeal extract and depression, 152
oatstraw, 124
Ockene, Dr. Judith and
physician misuse of hormones, 49
Women's Health Initiative, 49
olive oil, 103
onions, 110
organically grown food, 138
orgasm, 40–41
osteoporosis and
alcohol, 39
antidepressants, 38
bedrest/lack of exercise, 39
body fat, 39
caffeine, 39
calcium, 38
cigarette smoking, 39
environmental measures, 147–149
estrogen, 21
exercise, 169–170
herbs, 133–134
family history, 39
meat and animal products, 39
nutrition, 109–111
onions, 110
soy, 110
steroids, 39
stress reduction/healing, 192
thyroid/parathyroid hormones, 39
vitamin D, 38
ovaries and
estrogen, 20
menstruation, 20
progesterone, 20
"ovary failure," 8

pain busters, 167–168
palpitations and vitamin B12, 96–97
partial hysterectomy, 22
PCBs, 137
perimenopause and
a definition, 17
breast cancer, 28
cold hands, 28
complex carbohydrates, 107
hypothyroidism, 28
peppermint essential oil, 142
pesticides, 138
petrissage, 222
phthhalates, 141
phytoestrogen, 122
physician
communication style, 228
practice style, 227
Pick, M., OB/GYN nurse
practitioner and
bioidentical estradiol patch, 65
low-dose progesterone cream, 65
pine tar soap, 152
placebo, 36
pleasure points, 150
positive guided imagery, 179
postmenopause, 18
potassium and heart, 95
practitioner
appointments (preparing for), 234
certification, 230
checklist, 336–337
communication, 234
credentials, 230
disciplinary action, 230–231
experience, 230
hours, 231
race, 227
references, 231
referral, 229
screening, 231
similarity to other practitioners, 229